Body by Design

The Biohacker's Blueprint to Optimal Health

Written by Jon Ramsey
Published by Cornell-David Publishing House

Index

1. Introduction: The Biohacker's Journey to Optimal Health

The Biohacker's Journey to Optimal Health

In today's increasingly fast-paced and demanding world, people are more dedicated than ever to become their healthiest and best selves. Many individuals are turning to advancements in science, technology, and nutrition to unlock their true potential, transforming their bodies and minds to reach optimal health. This fascinating new paradigm, known as "biohacking," is a cutting-edge, multifaceted approach to self-improvement that involves tweaking and optimizing various aspects of lifestyle and biology.

Throughout history, humans have continuously strived to adapt and innovate to survive and thrive. The art and science of biohacking perfectly encapsulate this innate drive to push the boundaries of what's possible while remaining anchored in fundamental and scientific principles. In "Body by Design: The Biohacker's Blueprint to Optimal Health," we will delve deep into the world of biohacking, exploring groundbreaking ideas and techniques that can help you increase your energy, enhance your cognitive function, and support your overall well-being.

The Foundations of Biohacking

While everyone's biohacking journey may be unique, there are some foundational pillars that each individual should focus on to achieve optimal health. These pillars include nutrition, exercise, sleep, mindfulness, and technology. In the following sections, we will explore each of these in-depth along with the emerging science and technology that supports their integration into a comprehensive biohacking strategy.

Nutrition: Fueling the Body and Mind

"You are what you eat" might be an old adage, but it stands truer than ever in the realm of biohacking. Nutrient-dense foods serve as the fuel that powers our bodies and minds, and harnessing new breakthroughs in nutritional science can enable us to drive further improvements in physical and cognitive performance. In this section, we will discuss essential dietary considerations such as macronutrients, micronutrients, hydration, and supplementation. Additionally, we will explore trending dietary regimens, such as intermittent fasting, ketogenic diets, and plant-based living, along with their potential benefits and pitfalls.

Exercise: Building a Strong Body and Resilient Mind

Physical fitness is a critical component of overall health and well-being, closely linked to robust cardiovascular function, stress reduction, and mental sharpness. Biohacking the realm of exercise involves not only understanding how different forms of training can lead to better performance and physique but also learning how exercise impacts essential physiological processes such as metabolism, hormonal regulation, and neuroplasticity. This section will cover fundamental concepts of exercise science, introduce various training modalities such as high-intensity interval training (HIIT), resistance training, mobility work, and recovery techniques geared to help you enhance your biohacking journey.

Sleep: The Science of Rest and Recovery

A good night's sleep is the bedrock of health and well-being. Unfortunately, many people overlook its importance in our always-on, constantly connected world. Quality sleep is essential to cognitive function, emotional regulation, physical recovery, and immune system health. In this section, we will dive into the fascinating world of sleep science, exploring the vital role sleep plays in our health and performance, as well as providing practical, evidence-based tips to improve your sleep hygiene and optimize your wakefulness during the day.

Mindfulness: Cultivating Inner Balance and Clarity

The mind is an immensely powerful tool, capable of incredible feats of creativity, problem-solving, and awareness. In the pursuit of optimal health and performance, it's essential that we not only recognize the influence of our mental state on our overall health but actively cultivate practices that enhance inner balance and clarity. This section will introduce the science and practice of mindfulness, exploring techniques such as meditation, deep breathing, and visualization that can help you achieve greater mental harmony, increase focus, and reduce stress.

Technology: Harnessing New Tools for Health Optimization

As advancements in science and technology continue to change the landscape of health and wellness, biohackers have access to a plethora of new tools and data sources that can help to create a more nuanced and personalized approach to self-improvement. Wearable fitness trackers, genetic testing, and mobile applications are just a few examples of emerging technologies that can provide actionable insights to help us fine-tune our strategies and measure progress. This section will explore the latest gadgets, apps, and services available to biohackers and how to effectively implement them into your toolkit to optimize your overall health and well-being.

By carefully examining and applying the knowledge of these fundamental pillars, you will be well-equipped to embark on your biohacker's journey to optimal health. In "Body by Design: The Biohacker's Blueprint to Optimal Health," you will find not only inspiration but actionable guidance to transform your mind, body, and life on the way to unlocking new peaks of health, performance, and longevity.

Embracing the Biohacker's Mindset: Unlocking Your Personal Health Potential

To embark on the journey to optimal health, one must first understand and embrace the mindset of a biohacker. Biohacking, fundamentally, is the systematic approach to self-experimentation in order to optimize your mental and physical performance. By harnessing scientific knowledge, technology, nutrition, and various techniques, biohackers aim to take control of their bodies and minds to achieve peak performance.

The Science and the Art of Biohacking

Biohacking synergizes the principles of science and personal experimentation in a way that allows individuals to take charge of their health and wellbeing. At its core, biohacking is based on the belief that our bodies are highly adaptable systems capable of profound transformation when given the right conditions and stimuli.

From ancient practices of meditation and fasting to cutting-edge research in genomics and neurobiology, biohackers fuse time-tested wisdom with scientific rigor to achieve optimal wellness.

Developing a Strong Foundation: Mindset and Habits

A critical element in the biohacker's journey is developing a mindset that prioritizes lifelong learning and experimentation. This requires consistently nurturing curiosity, adaptability, and resilience. Biohackers face the challenge of accepting changes in belief systems as new scientific evidence emerges, while remaining vigilant against pseudoscience and overhyped trends.

The cultivation of good habits — in terms of sleep quality, nutrition, exercise, stress management, and mental wellbeing — is the bedrock upon which sustained success in biohacking rests. Disciplined routines, mindfulness practices, and self-reflection enable a biohacker to fine-tune their strategies for peak performance continuously.

Self-Quantification: Measuring What Matters

Collecting and analyzing data about one's biological systems is a hallmark of biohacking. With the rise of wearable devices, personalized health tracking apps, and direct-to-consumer genetic testing, biohackers are increasingly leveraging data-driven insights to customize their health and wellness routines.

Analyzing metrics for sleep, stress, cognitive performance, physical activity, and health biomarkers can help biohackers identify both strengths and weaknesses in their approach. This information is invaluable when refining interventions and adjusting strategies to better support individual needs and goals.

Navigating the Biohacking Toolbox: Techniques and Technologies

Armed with an open, curious mindset and a strong foundation of data-driven self-awareness, the biohacker can begin exploring the wealth of diverse tools, techniques, and technologies available for optimizing their personal health and performance.

This broad toolbox includes:

- Nutrition and supplementation strategies like intermittent fasting, ketogenic diets, and nootropics.
- Exercise and movement practices such as high-intensity interval training (HIIT), yoga, or functional fitness.
- Sleep and stress management techniques, including meditation, mindfulness exercises, and smart sleep trackers.
- Cognitive enhancement approaches, encompassing brain training tools, neurofeedback, and transcranial magnetic stimulation.

- Advanced biological interventions like genome editing, cellular reprogramming, or stem cell therapy.

It is essential to understand that not all methods will benefit everyone equally, given the uniqueness of our individual genetic and environmental factors. Adopting a rigorous scientific mindset, biohackers must experiment, observe, and adjust their health strategies according to their specific needs, goals, and responses.

Connecting the Dots: Biohacking as a Holistic Approach to Optimal Health

Central to the biohacking mindset is a recognition that health and wellness are not a collection of isolated processes but are instead part of an interconnected web of systems within the body. As such, biohackers seek to optimize on a holistic level, intertwining their efforts in nutrition, exercise, sleep, mental health, and cutting-edge technologies to support the entire body's ability to adapt, grow, and thrive.

By integrating diverse approaches to health and functioning, biohacking enables individuals to map their unique journey to optimal wellbeing, empowering them to take control of their biology and harness untapped potential. This journey, while often challenging, ultimately leads to a state of profound self-mastery, where the biohacker can experience peak physical, cognitive, and emotional performance.

Understanding the Biohacker's Journey to Optimal Health

Before we dive into the world of biohacking, it's crucial to understand the core principles that underlie this cutting-edge approach to health, wellness, and performance optimization. From gaining mental clarity for peak productivity, to leveraging biological processes in our favor, the journey to biohacking success rests upon our ability to develop effective and personalized strategies based on our own biological make-up.

A. Embracing the Mindset of the Biohacker

Biohacking, at its core, is a do-it-yourself (DIY) approach to understanding and optimizing human biology. By breaking down our bodies, behaviors, and habits into their most fundamental components, biohackers can make more informed decisions about how to improve their health and thrive in their daily lives.

Three critical elements define the biohacker's mindset:

1. **Curiosity**: Biohackers possess an insatiable desire to learn, explore, and understand how their bodies respond to various inputs, be it nutrition, exercise, sleep, or technology. Curiosity is both an innate trait and a muscle to be flexed, allowing individuals to uncover new avenues for self-improvement.
2. **Self-Experimentation**: Long-term success in the world of biohacking comes from intentional trial and error, relentless testing of oneself, and being open to learning from personal experiences. By developing a hypothesis, testing possible solutions, and adapting based on the results, biohackers can make systematic progress towards their health goals.
3. **Resilience**: Biohackers can expect to encounter obstacles on their journey, from setbacks in personal progress to failed experiments. What sets successful biohackers apart from others is the ability to persevere through these challenges, drawing valuable

insights from each step of the process and using them to move forward.

B. Leveraging Scientific Insights for Personal Advantage

The success of biohacking initiatives relies heavily on the application and integration of modern scientific research. By understanding the principles behind various biological processes, biohackers can confidently align their practices with empirical evidence, ensuring that their endeavors are based on solid foundations.

As we move through this book, we will break down complex scientific concepts, discuss their relevance to the biohacker's journey, and prescribe actionable steps to apply them to our daily lives.

C. Establishing Holistic Goals

A goal-oriented approach is central to the biohacker's blueprint, but it's important to remember that this is not a one-size-fits-all process. Each individual will possess unique strengths, weaknesses, and objectives, making it critical for biohackers to establish tailored goals in order to optimize their health holistically.

When setting these goals, consider the different dimensions of health: physical, mental, emotional, and spiritual. Strive to create SMART (Specific, Measurable, Attainable, Relevant, and Time-sensitive) objectives that align with your personal values and aspirations, allowing you to recognize your progress and maintain motivation.

D. Navigating the World of Biohacking Tools and Technologies

As biohackers, we live in an exciting era, with new tools and technologies emerging at a rapid pace. From wearables that track sleep and heart rate variability to apps that offer meditation and cognitive training exercises, the possibilities are vast. We will explore these tools throughout the book and discuss how they can be used to complement and enhance the biohacker's journey.

By incorporating cutting-edge technologies into our biohacking toolbox, we can collect valuable data, set quantifiable targets, and effectively monitor our progress on the road to optimal health.

E. The Power of Community

Biohacking may be a personal journey, but it does not need to be a solitary one. The biohacking community is a global network of individuals seeking to improve their health and the collective understanding of human biology. By engaging with like-minded individuals, sharing experiences, and celebrating successes, biohackers can maintain accountability, glean insights from others' experiences, and bolster their motivation.

Throughout this book, we will discuss strategies for forging meaningful connections with fellow biohackers, both online and offline, and learning from the vibrant community of thinkers and doers propelling the movement forward.

Together, these five themes provide a holistic framework for the biohacker's journey to optimal health. By embracing the mindset, leveraging scientific insights, aligning with personal goals, incorporating innovative tools, and fostering community connections, you will be well set up to succeed on your own journey.

In the following chapters, we will delve into the fascinating world of biohacking, exploring specific practices, tips, and principles to help you create a lifestyle that supports your ultimate health, wellness, and personal success. Welcome to the fascinating world of Body by Design. Your journey to optimal health starts now.

1.1 The New Frontier: Biohacking Your Body

Welcome to the brave new world of biohacking, where innovative thinkers and passionate individuals are re-defining the boundaries of human performance, health, and well-being. By leveraging the power of science, technology, and self-experimentation, biohackers are unlocking the secrets to optimizing our physical, mental, and emotional states. This journey of self-discovery is opening up an entirely new frontier of possibilities for attaining peak performance and longevity.

1.1.1 What is Biohacking?

At its core, biohacking is the practice of modifying and improving our biological systems using a range of techniques and tools. These methods range from simple dietary changes, exercise, and sleep hygiene to more advanced technologies such as wearables, nootropics, and genetic engineering. The goal of biohacking is to optimize our bodies and minds, enabling us to lead healthier, more productive lives.

As biohackers, we are not content to simply accept the status quo of our biology. We believe in the potential of the human body to evolve and adapt, and we are driven to push the boundaries of what it means to be human. By experimenting and iterating on our bodies and minds, we are forging a path towards a brighter, healthier future.

1.1.2 The Biohacker's Toolbox

The world of biohacking is vast and varied, and as such, there are many different tools and techniques that you may encounter on your journey. Some of the most common biohacking methods include:

1. **Nutrition**: One of the fundamental aspects of biohacking is optimizing our diets to ensure that our bodies are receiving the nutrients they need to function at their best. By tweaking our diets, we can give ourselves the energy required to power through the day, support our cognitive functions, and increase our overall health and well-being.
2. **Exercise**: Regular physical activity is a crucial aspect of biohacking, as it not only contributes to better cardiovascular health but also helps to maintain a healthy body composition, increase focus, and promote overall well-being.
3. **Sleep**: Optimizing sleep is an essential cornerstone of any biohacking endeavor, as it plays a crucial role in our mood, cognitive abilities, and overall health. By improving the quality and duration of our sleep, we can maximize the restorative benefits of this essential process.
4. **Stress Management**: Effective stress management is another vital aspect of biohacking, as chronic stress can have detrimental effects on our physical and emotional health. Incorporating mindfulness practices

and other stress-reduction techniques into our daily routines can help us better handle the inevitable stressors of life.

5. **Supplements & Nootropics**: Biohackers may experiment with a wide range of supplements and nootropics in order to augment their cognitive and physical performance. These substances can include vitamins, minerals, herbal extracts, and other compounds that are believed to support optimal health.

6. **Wearables & Technology**: A variety of technological tools and devices can be employed in the service of biohacking, from fitness trackers and smartwatches that monitor our physical activities and biometrics to advanced neuro-tech devices that stimulate brain function and improve cognitive abilities.

7. **Environmental Modifications**: Biohackers often make subtle adjustments to their surroundings to promote optimal health and well-being. Examples include optimizing the indoor air quality in their living spaces, adjusting lighting to promote healthy circadian rhythms, and creating ergonomic workspaces that promote good posture and mitigate the risk of injury.

1.1.3 The Biohacker's Mindset

At the heart of biohacking lies a deep-seated curiosity about the workings of the human body and an unwavering commitment to self-improvement. As such, many biohackers adopt a growth mindset, viewing their bodies and minds as malleable systems that can be continuously upgraded and refined.

One of the key tenets of the biohacker's mindset is the practice of self-experimentation. While there is a wealth of information and research available to inform our biohacking efforts, each individual's biology is unique, and as such, personal experimentation is crucial in order to determine the most effective strategies for our specific needs.

This spirit of experimentation extends beyond the confines of our individual biology, as biohackers are driven to share their findings and breakthroughs with the wider community. By pooling our knowledge and exchanging experiences, we can accelerate the pace of discovery and potentially unlock new frontiers in human health and performance.

1.1.4 Navigating the Biohacker's Journey

Embarking on the biohacker's journey can seem intimidating at first, with its myriad of techniques, terminology, and technology. However, this blueprint aims to provide a comprehensive guide and resource for those who wish to begin or continue their journey towards optimal health.

As you delve deeper into the world of biohacking, keep in mind that progress is rarely linear, and setbacks are an inevitable part of the process. Remember to approach each experiment and modification with an open mind, and be prepared to learn from both your successes and challenges.

In the end, the journey is just as important as the destination – and we are here to support you every step of the way. Together, we can unlock the transformative potential of biohacking and create a future where we all have the opportunity to thrive.

A New Era of Personalized Health Optimization: The Biohacker's Path to Wellness

As the sun rises on a new era of health and wellness, marked by the unprecedented advancements made in the realms of genetics, technology, and nutrition, a community of individuals passionate about understanding and manipulating the human body's potential has come together, forging the path to optimal health: Biohacking.

The term biohacking combines *"biology"* (the science of living organisms) with *"hacking"* (finding shortcuts, workarounds, or novel ways to solve complex problems). Broadly construed, biohacking refers to an ongoing exploration of the human body and mind, with the ultimate goal of optimizing physical and cognitive performance. In essence, biohackers are "health hackers" who experiment with a diverse range of modalities, technologies, and lifestyle changes to unlock peak wellbeing.

Biohacking represents an exciting new chapter in one's personal journey towards optimal health. By treating the body as a complex system of interconnected components, biohackers develop an awareness of the various ways in which these individual components can be augmented or adjusted, leading to the potential for profound transformations in health, cognition, and overall performance.

In this introductory section, we will lay the groundwork for the biohacking journey, offering an overview of the major domains within which biohackers operate, the tools and technologies they employ to pursue their goals, and the principles that guide their collective approach to achieving peak health.

Core Domains of Biohacking

Biohacking can be broken down into several core domains, each focusing on specific aspects of the human system and how they can be fine-tuned to achieve optimal health:

1. **Nutrition** - Biohackers embrace a systems-based approach to understanding how the food we consume interacts with our unique biochemistry. Food becomes fuel, medicine, and a tool for enhancing physical performance and cognitive functioning.
2. **Exercise** - Biohackers emphasize the importance of movement and the role it plays in enhancing body composition, optimizing organ function, and promoting overall well-being. They employ science-backed exercise strategies that yield maximal results with minimal time investment.
3. **Sleep** - This crucial component of our daily lives is often overlooked, but biohackers recognize the power of quality sleep in promoting optimal physical and mental performance. Hacking sleep involves understanding personal sleep patterns, mastering the sleep environment, and employing techniques to achieve deeper and more restorative sleep.
4. **Stress Management** - Chronic stress can wreak havoc on our bodies and minds. Biohackers develop personalized strategies for reducing stress levels and enhancing resilience, using practices such as mindfulness and self-care to radically improve wellbeing.
5. **Cognitive Enhancement** - Unlocking the potential of the brain is a key endeavor in the biohacking community. Cognitive enhancement involves using

various tools, technologies, and practices designed to improve memory, focus, creativity, and other cognitive functions.
6. **Technology** - From wearable devices to cutting-edge biofeedback systems, technology is an essential component of the biohacking toolkit. Leveraging these innovations presents opportunities to gather data, analyze personal health metrics, and develop targeted interventions for achieving optimal health and performance.

Biohacking Principles: A Holistic Approach to Health

As disparate as these domains may appear, they are united by a set of core principles that underpin the biohacking philosophy:

1. **Personalization** - One size does not fit all. Each person's body is unique, and successful biohacking requires a personalized approach based on individual genetics, lifestyle, and preferences.
2. **Self-experimentation** - The biohacking journey is driven by curiosity and experimentation. Biohackers are not afraid to tinker with their bodies, fine-tuning various inputs and measuring the effects to identify the most effective strategies for optimization.
3. **Pragmatism** - Biohackers are driven by results, not dogma. The focus is on finding what works best through trial and error and adopting an open-minded approach to health and wellness.
4. **Evidence-based practice** - Biohacking derives its power from the scientific method, relying on evidence to discern which interventions produce real, measurable, and sustainable results.

5. **Community** - Biohackers come from diverse backgrounds, but are united by a shared passion for understanding and optimizing the human body. We learn from one another and share knowledge, creating a powerful global network of biohackers committed to achieving optimal health.

With a strong foundation in these domains and principles, the biohacker's journey to optimal health presents numerous opportunities for growth, exploration, and personal transformation. As we delve further into "Body by Design: The Biohacker's Blueprint to Optimal Health," we invite you to join us in unlocking your full potential and reclaiming the vibrant health and wellbeing that is your birthright. Together, we will continue to push the boundaries of human potential, transcending limitations and redefining the meaning of true health and happiness.

2. The Mind-Body Connection: Harnessing Neuroscience for Peak Performance

2.1 Understanding The Mind-Body Connection: The Power of Neuroscience

The mind-body connection is a fascinating and multi-faceted concept that has gained increasing prominence in recent years. This deeper understanding of how our bodies and minds are interconnected at a molecular level has ultimately enabled us to harness neuroscience for peak performance in every aspect of our lives. Let's take a deeper dive into the fascinating world of the mind-body connection and explore some strategies to optimize our cognitive and physical functioning.

The Science Behind the Mind-Body Connection

Neuroscience is the study of the nervous system, which includes the brain, spinal cord, and peripheral nerves. This complex network allows for the communication of information between all areas of the body and directly influences our experiences, emotions, thoughts, and actions. In essence, the mind-body connection is rooted in the intricate interplay between these various components of the nervous system.

Notably, this synergistic relationship relies on a of series chemical messengers known as neurotransmitters. These molecules transmit information throughout the brain and body, orchestrating a symphony of functions that influence everything from our mood to our metabolism. For example, serotonin, a neurotransmitter often associated with mood regulation, can also influence our appetite and digestion. It becomes unmistakably clear that optimizing our neurochemistry is essential for maintaining overall equilibrium within our bodies.

Biohacking Your Brain: Strategies to Optimize Cognitive Function

Achieving peak mental performance is a cornerstone of the biohacker's blueprint, as it underpins our ability to fully harness the power of our mind-body connection. Here are some proven strategies to support optimal cognitive function:

- **Sleep Optimization**: Sleep is crucial for the rejuvenation and repair of the brain, as well as memory consolidation and emotional processing. Aim for 7-9 hours of quality sleep each night and prioritize a consistent sleep-wake schedule.

- **Nutrition**: A brain-healthy diet should be rich in omega-3 fatty acids, antioxidants, vitamins, and minerals. Consider incorporating anti-inflammatory foods, such as leafy greens, nuts, and fatty fish, as well as brain-boosting supplements like curcumin and magnesium.
- **Exercise**: Regular physical activity has been shown to improve cognitive function, increase brain volume, and even create new brain cells. Aim for a mix of moderate-to-vigorous aerobic exercise, strength training, and mind-body practices like yoga.
- **Meditation and Mindfulness**: Techniques like meditation and deep breathing can help to increase awareness, focus, and self-regulation, promoting overall mental well-being. Regular practice can help to reduce stress and regulate mood by modulating neurotransmitter function.
- **Neurofeedback**: This cutting-edge biohacking tool allows individuals to monitor and modify their brainwave patterns in real-time. By adjusting these patterns, it becomes possible to optimize cognitive performance, mood, and overall brain function.

Tapping into the Somatic Power of the Mind-Body Connection

The mind-body connection reaches beyond cognitive function, also encompassing the somatic experience of our bodies. This means that our thoughts, emotions, and stress levels all have an undeniable impact on our physical health. Embracing this notion, let's explore some approaches to managing stress and emotions for peak physical performance:

- **Emotional Freedom Technique (EFT)**: Also known as "tapping," EFT is a non-invasive technique involving gentle pressure applied to specific acupressure points on the body. The goal is to stimulate these energy pathways to release blocked emotions, thereby reducing stress and anxiety.
- **Breathwork**: Controlled breathing exercises can help to activate the parasympathetic nervous system, which induces a state of restfulness and promotes recovery. There are many approaches to breathwork, including slow diaphragmatic breathing, box breathing, and alternate nostril breathing.
- **Grounding**: Reconnecting with nature is a powerful way to harness the mind-body connection. Grounding, also known as "earthing," is the act of making direct contact with the earth's surface, which is believed to promote balance and reduce inflammation throughout the body.
- **Biofeedback**: By using various devices, biofeedback enables us to gain insight into our physiological responses and consciously control them. Popular forms of biofeedback include heart rate variability (HRV) training and muscle tension monitoring.

In conclusion, the mind-body connection is the fundamental underpinning of optimal health and well-being. By understanding the science of this connection and adopting various strategies to support our brain and body, we can achieve peak performance in every aspect of our lives. As the realm of neuroscience continues to expand, biohackers are at the forefront of advancing our understanding and harnessing the incredible power of the mind-body connection.

2.1 Understanding the Neuroscience of Mind-Body Connection

The mind-body connection has been an area of growing interest and research, as it can play a fundamental role in enhancing our well-being and overall performance. This connection signifies the powerful interdependence of our mental and emotional states on our physical health, and vice versa. Understanding the principles of neuroscience and the mechanisms behind the mind-body connection can help biohackers optimize their health, emphasizing not only fitness but also emotional resilience and cognitive flexibility.

2.1.1 The Basics of Neuroscience

Neuroscience is the scientific study of the nervous system, which comprises the brain, spinal cord, and nerves that are distributed throughout the body. It focuses on understanding the structure and function of these neural networks, how they process information and ultimately govern all aspects of our behavior, cognition, and emotions.

In recent years, thanks to rapid advancements in technology and non-invasive imaging techniques such as functional magnetic resonance imaging (fMRI), researchers have been able to closely observe and measure brain activity. Through these advances, we are continually expanding our knowledge of the intricate connections between our thoughts, feelings, and bodily responses.

2.1.2 The Role of Neurotransmitters in the Mind-Body Connection

One of the primary ways our brain and body communicate are through neurotransmitters. These are chemical messengers that transmit signals across synapses, or gaps between neurons, to facilitate communication and relay information throughout the nervous system. They play a crucial role in regulating a wide range of bodily functions, including mood, appetite, sleep, pain perception, muscle movement, and even learning and memory.

Some of the key neurotransmitters that influence our mind-body connection include:

- **Serotonin**: Known as the "feel-good" neurotransmitter, serotonin contributes to feelings of happiness, well-being, and contentment. It also helps regulate sleep, appetite, and cognitive function.
- **Dopamine**: This neurotransmitter is associated with feelings of pleasure and reward, as well as motivation and attention.
- **Norepinephrine**: Often referred to as adrenaline, norepinephrine is responsible for our fight-or-flight response in the face of stress or danger. It increases alertness, heart rate, and blood pressure.
- **Endorphins**: These natural opioids are released in response to pain, exercise, or other forms of stress, evoking feelings of euphoria and working as natural painkillers.
- **GABA (Gamma-Aminobutyric Acid)**: GABA is an inhibitory neurotransmitter that helps calm the nervous system, promoting relaxation and reducing anxiety.

By influencing these neurotransmitters through targeted interventions and biohacks, we can modulate our emotions, enhance our physical performance, and ultimately boost our overall well-being.

2.1.3 The Impact of Stress on the Mind-Body Connection

It's essential to recognize the role of stress in the mind-body connection, as chronic stress can wreak havoc on both our mental and physical health. When we experience stress or perceive a threat, our brain activates the hypothalamic-pituitary-adrenal (HPA) axis, a complex network of communication that releases various hormones into the bloodstream, including cortisol.

Cortisol, the primary stress hormone, triggers the body's fight-or-flight response, diverting energy toward essential systems and functions, such as our heart rate, blood pressure, and muscle activation. While this response is generally adaptive in the face of short-term stress, chronic stress can lead to elevated cortisol levels, which can have detrimental effects on our health, including:

- Suppressed immune system
- Increased blood pressure
- Weight gain, particularly around the abdomen
- Mood disorders, such as anxiety and depression
- Memory impairment and cognitive decline

As biohackers, understanding our stress responses and working to mitigate them or channel them productively is crucial in maintaining an optimized mind-body connection.

2.1.4 Biohacking Techniques for Enhanced Mind-Body Connection

Integrating the principles of neuroscience and understanding the mind-body connection offers a range of biohacking techniques and strategies to enhance our overall fitness, emotional resilience, and cognitive performance. Some of these techniques include:

1. **Meditation**: Practicing mindfulness meditation can help increase our awareness of both our thoughts and bodily sensations, ultimately fostering a stronger mind-body connection. Research has shown that meditation can reduce stress, improve focus, and enhance emotional well-being.
2. **Nutrition**: Consuming a well-balanced diet rich in nutrients, vitamins, and minerals is crucial for optimal neurotransmitter synthesis and function. Ensuring adequate levels of mood-boosting nutrients such as omega-3 fatty acids, tryptophan, and antioxidants can support both brain health and overall wellness.
3. **Exercise**: Engaging in regular physical activity can enhance the release of endorphins, serotonin, and other beneficial neurotransmitters, promoting stress reduction, improved mood, and increased cognitive function.
4. **Sleep**: Prioritizing sleep is of utmost importance, as it plays a vital role in regulating our neurotransmitters and maintaining the delicate balance of our mind-body connection. Practicing good sleep hygiene and establishing a consistent sleep routine can help support optimal brain function and overall health.
5. **Social Connection**: Establishing and maintaining healthy social connections is vital for both mental and physical health. Research has shown that a strong social support network can help buffer against the negative impacts of stress and improve overall well-being.

In conclusion, understanding and harnessing the power of the mind-body connection through the lens of neuroscience can act as a powerful tool for biohackers seeking to optimize their health, performance, and overall well-being. By engaging in targeted interventions that modulate neurotransmitter levels, reduce stress, and facilitate a stronger connection between our minds and bodies, we can create the most favorable internal environment for peak performance and resilience in the face of life's inevitable challenges.

Unlocking the Power of Neuroplasticity: Rewiring Your Brain for Success

One of the most groundbreaking developments in contemporary neuroscience is our ever-increasing understanding of neuroplasticity — the brain's remarkable ability to reorganize, adapt, and rewire itself throughout our lives. Utilizing the principles of neuroplasticity, we can accelerate our mental and physical transformation by actively reshaping our neural pathways and optimizing our cognitive functioning. From enhancing memory to amplifying focus, the following practices can empower you to develop a truly high-performance brain and unlock your full cognitive potential.

Brain Training: Stimulating Neurogenesis & Synaptic Strengthening

Contrary to popular belief, our brains never actually cease growing and evolving. Recent research has shown that the neurons in our brains continuously form new connections and regenerate in a phenomenon known as neurogenesis. To bolster and maintain this process, several strategies can be employed.

Cognitive Exercises

Just as physical exercise keeps our bodies fit, cognitive exercises help sharpen our mental abilities. Problems that require complex reasoning, planning, and strategizing, like logic puzzles, spatial visualization tests or riddles, can help stretch our brains by demanding neurological fitness. Further, learning new skills or engaging in novel activities can stimulate the production of new neurons and improve neural interconnectivity. For instance, try learning a foreign language, mastering a musical instrument, or engaging in a new hobby to keep your brain sharp and youthful.

Balanced Sleep & Relaxation

Numerous studies have shown that getting sufficient sleep is critical for promoting neurogenesis and maintaining optimal cognitive performance. Aim for at least 7-8 hours of sleep per night, ensuring you pass through all crucial sleep stages, including the restorative REM cycle. Additionally, partaking in regular relaxation and mindfulness practices, such as meditation, can not only help manage stress levels but also improve cognitive functioning.

Boosting Neurotransmitter Production for Enhanced Focus & Motivation

Neurotransmitters are essential chemical messengers that transmit signals throughout our neural networks. Two main neurotransmitters, dopamine and norepinephrine, are responsible for regulating our focus, motivation, and overall sense of well-being. While some decline in transmitter production is natural with age, strategic lifestyle adjustments and supplementation can help restore optimal levels.

Diet & Lifestyle Optimization

Supporting healthy neurotransmitter production primarily starts with our diet. Ensuring that you consume substantial amounts of essential amino acids and other neurotransmitter precursors is crucial. Focus on protein-rich foods like fish, poultry, legumes, and dairy, and aim to include plenty of fruits, vegetables, and whole grains.

Additionally, make certain to engage in regular physical movement, be it through dedicated exercise sessions or by incorporating more movement into your daily life. Regular physical activity has been proven to increase the production of critical neurotransmitters, like serotonin, which can improve mood and alleviate anxiety.

Targeted Supplementation

Certain natural supplements can further support neurotransmitter synthesis and maintenance. A well-balanced multivitamin containing essential vitamins like B-complex, vitamins C and D, as well as minerals like magnesium and zinc, can help support optimal neural communications. Moreover, specific amino acid supplements such as L-tyrosine and L-tryptophan may be utilized to promote the production of key neurotransmitters such as dopamine and serotonin.

Mindfulness & Stress Reduction: Elevating Cognitive Performance

Chronic stress can wreak havoc on our brains and diminish overall cognitive functioning. Actively addressing stress and cultivating a more balanced, mindful state of being can profoundly improve our capacity for creative thinking and problem-solving.

Meditation & Breathwork

Cultivating a regular meditation practice, even as little as 10-20 minutes per day, can not only help reduce stress levels but also increase the thickness of the prefrontal cortex, which is responsible for higher-order cognitive functions like attention, decision-making, and self-regulation. In addition, breathwork exercises, such as deep diaphragmatic breathing or alternate nostril breathing, can help lower cortisol levels, promoting a relaxed mental state and improved cognitive performance.

Mindset Training

Nurturing a positive, growth-oriented mindset is essential in combating the forces of self-doubt, anxiety, and negativity. Techniques like visualization, affirmations, and journaling can help maintain a more balanced mind and enhance your performance in various aspects of your life.

In conclusion, by taking a proactive approach to your mental well-being and employing proven neuroscientific techniques, you can unlock your brain's tremendous potential for success. Embrace the power of neuroplasticity and transform your cognitive capacities, paving the way for a life of vibrant health, peak performance, and limitless possibilities.

2.1 Understanding the Neuroscience of Peak Performance

A critical aspect of biohacking is understanding the role of the brain and the nervous system in achieving peak performance. In this section, we will explore the core components of the neuroscience of optimal performance and provide a guide on harnessing these powerful tools to help you achieve your goals.

2.1.1 The Central Role of the Brain in Peak Performance

Before we delve deeper into the neuroscience of peak performance, it is essential to understand the role the brain plays in controlling our physical and mental transformations. The brain is the master regulator of our body, responsible for coordinating and integrating all our physiological systems. It also serves as 'mission control' for our thoughts, emotions, and behavior patterns.

Achieving peak performance is predicated on optimal brain function. At the core of this process is our brain's ability to process information, make decisions, focus attention, and regulate emotions. As such, biohackers must gain a thorough understanding of the brain-to-body connection and employ strategies that facilitate improvements in overall brain health and cognitive function.

2.1.2 Elements of the Neuroscience of Peak Performance

Several key elements of neuroscience contribute to our understanding of peak performance. These elements include neuroplasticity, neural efficiency, neuromodulation, neurogenesis, and neuroprotective factors. By harnessing the power of these elements, biohackers can set the stage for unleashing their full physical and mental potential.

- **Neuroplasticity**: This component refers to the brain's ability to adapt and change throughout life continually. Neurons (brain cells) can form new connections and pathways, allowing the brain to reorganize itself in response to new experiences, learning, and injury. Harnessing neuroplasticity can facilitate improvements in cognitive and physical performance.
- **Neural efficiency**: Neural efficiency is the capacity of the brain to use the least possible amount of energy to perform a task effectively. A more efficient brain means better cognitive performance and a greater ability to focus attention on the task at hand, as well as faster response times and problem-solving capabilities.
- **Neuromodulation**: Neuromodulation involves the release of various neurotransmitters and other molecules that modulate the activity of neurons throughout the brain. Some key neurotransmitters involved in peak performance include dopamine (for motivation, focus, and reward processing), serotonin (for mood, appetite, and impulse control), and norepinephrine (for alertness, attention, and energy). Optimizing the levels and functioning of these neuromodulators is essential for achieving peak performance in both mental and physical domains.
- **Neurogenesis**: Neurogenesis refers to the process by which new neurons are formed in the brain. By promoting new neuronal growth, biohackers can stimulate improvements in memory, learning, and cognitive function.

- **Neuroprotective factors**: These are substances that help to protect the brain from damage and maintain proper brain health. Some examples include antioxidants, which can mitigate oxidative stress, and growth factors such as brain-derived neurotrophic factor (BDNF), which supports the survival of existing neurons and promotes the growth and development of new ones.

2.1.3 Strategies for Harnessing Neuroscience in Biohacking

In order to effectively harness the power of neuroscience for peak performance, biohackers must adopt a holistic approach that incorporates various lifestyle factors, nutrition, exercise, and supplementation. These strategies are designed to foster optimal brain health and cognitive function, as well as overall physiological wellbeing.

- **Lifestyle modifications**: Some core lifestyle factors that have been shown to influence brain health and cognitive function include sleep, stress management, and social engagement. By optimizing your sleep patterns, managing stress through techniques such as meditation or mindfulness, and engaging in meaningful social interactions, you can promote better brain health and cognitive function.
- **Nutrition**: A diet rich in nutrients that support brain health and cognitive function is essential for peak performance. Some key nutritional components include omega-3 fatty acids, antioxidants, and B-vitamins. In addition, emphasizing a diet rich in whole foods, and low in processed and sugary foods, can help reduce inflammation and provide the brain with the necessary building blocks for optimal function.

- **Exercise**: Regular physical activity is known to have a multitude of benefits for brain health and cognitive function. Exercise promotes the release of BDNF and other growth factors, enhances neuroplasticity, and boosts overall mood and energy levels. A combination of aerobic exercise, such as running or swimming, and resistance training can help promote optimal brain function and peak performance.
- **Supplementation**: Targeted supplementation with key nutrients and compounds that promote brain health and cognitive function can be a valuable addition to your biohacking toolkit. Nootropics, also known as 'smart drugs' or cognitive enhancers, can enhance memory, focus, creativity, and overall brain performance. Some examples of nootropics include caffeine, L-theanine, and adaptogenic herbs like Ashwagandha or Rhodiola Rosea. As with any supplementation regimen, be sure to consult with a healthcare professional to ensure safety and efficacy in your specific context.

By incorporating these strategies into your biohacking regimen, you will not only support overall brain health but also set the stage for peak performance in both mental and physical domains. As with any biohacking endeavor, remember that achieving optimal performance will take time and dedication; so be patient, stay persistent, and trust that your efforts will yield the desired results.

2.5 Hacking the Reward System: Dopamine, Biofeedback, and Neuroplasticity

The intricate connection between our mind and body serves as a basis for biohacking techniques aimed at improving not just our mental performance, but also our overall well-being. In this chapter, we will focus on understanding how the brain's reward system works, and how we can hack this system using the principles of biofeedback and neuroplasticity for peak performance.

2.5.1 Dopamine: The Neurotransmitter of Reward and Motivation

Dopamine is a major neurotransmitter within the brain, which acts as a signaling molecule responsible for the communication between neurons. It plays a key role in modulating various aspects of our brain function, the most notable of which is the reward system. The reward system is an evolutionary development that helps us seek pleasurable experiences and engage in behaviors we find rewarding. When we achieve a goal or receive positive feedback, our brain's reward system is triggered, and dopamine is released within the nucleus accumbens, a key brain region linked with pleasure and reward.

In essence, dopamine fuels motivation, drives decision-making, and shapes our behavior through feelings of pleasure and satisfaction. Understanding how the dopamine system works can provide valuable insights into hacking this "reward chemical" to optimize performance, motivation, and mental well-being.

2.5.2 Biofeedback: Listening to the Language of Your Body

Biofeedback is a mind-body technique that teaches individuals how to gain control over various physiological functions, such as heart rate, blood pressure, and muscle tension. By monitoring these functions through electronic instruments, biofeedback enables individuals to receive real-time feedback on their physiological state. With this newfound awareness, individuals can then manipulate their physiological responses and consequently, modify their thoughts, emotions, and behaviors.

To make the connection with dopamine and the reward system, biofeedback can help us become more attuned to the signals our body sends us, enabling us to reinforce positive outcomes and curb negative ones. For example, wearing a heart-rate monitor during exercise allows us to adapt our workout pace and intensity to maintain an optimal heart rate, thereby capitalizing on the release of dopamine and other performance-enhancing neurotransmitters. The more we practice biofeedback techniques, the more skilled we become at recognizing our body's cues and adjusting our responses accordingly.

2.5.3 Neuroplasticity: Shaping the Brain through Experience

Neuroplasticity, or the ability of the brain to change and adapt in response to various experiences and stimuli, lies at the heart of our capacity for personal growth and development. Through understanding the principles of neuroplasticity, we can harness our brain's plastic nature to reshape neural pathways and circuits, ultimately improving our mental performance and contributing to peak performance.

The process of neuroplasticity can be divided into two subtypes - synaptic plasticity and structural plasticity. Synaptic plasticity refers to the alterations in the strength and connections of synapses (the junctions where two neurons communicate), while structural plasticity involves the formation of entirely new neurons, a phenomenon known as neurogenesis. To alter these connections, we must repeatedly engage in the desired behavior or expose ourselves to specific stimuli, triggering neuroplastic adjustments over time.

One revolutionary way to harness neuroplasticity is through the use of neurofeedback, a form of biofeedback that directly targets the brain. Neurofeedback involves monitoring the brain's electrical activity via electroencephalography (EEG) and providing real-time feedback on brainwave patterns to the individual. By teaching individuals how to consciously regulate their brainwave patterns, they can learn to optimize their brain function and achieve desired cognitive states.

2.5.4 Practical Applications: Hacking Your Reward System for Peak Performance

The power of these techniques lies in their ability to address the underlying neural mechanisms associated with motivation, reward, and performance. Here are some practical applications to integrate into your biohacking routine:

1. **Set specific, achievable goals:** Research has shown that achieving small, well-defined tasks leads to a more substantial dopamine release as opposed to vague and distant goals. Break down your objectives into small, manageable tasks to optimize your motivation and leverage the power of dopamine release.
2. **Create a reward system:** Identify activities or experiences that stimulate the release of dopamine, such as desirable food or your favorite hobbies. Reward yourself with these activities after completing

a task to reinforce positive behavior and capitalize on the brain's reward system.

3. **Adopt mindfulness practices:** Techniques such as meditation and deep breathing exercises can help in reducing stress and promoting relaxation, which in turn supports a healthy dopamine response. Regular mindfulness practices help in keeping the dopamine receptors in the brain functioning optimally, ensuring an efficient reward system.

4. **Invest in neurofeedback sessions:** Although neurofeedback may initially seem like a complex and costly venture, it could be worth the investment in the long run. Engaging in regular neurofeedback training can lead to lasting neuroplastic changes that improve cognitive function, focus, and overall mental performance.

By gaining insights into the function of dopamine within our brain's reward system and leveraging the power of biofeedback and neuroplasticity techniques, we can effectively hack the mind-body connection to achieve personal growth, optimal cognitive function, and peak performance. With consistent practice and a commitment to self-improvement, soon enough, you will be well on your way to unlocking your full potential and becoming a true biohacker.

3. Nutritional Mastery: Personalizing Your Diet for Genetic Success

3.1 Understanding Your Genetic Makeup: How your genes impact your nutrition

Each individual has a unique genetic makeup, which makes it important to personalize your diet in order to maximize your genetic potential and reach optimal health. In recent years, significant advances in genomics research have expanded our understanding of the relationship between our genes, the nutrients we consume, and the overall impact on our health. Scientists have begun to unravel the complexities of how our DNA responds to and is influenced by foods, lifestyle choices, and our surroundings.

In this section, we will discuss the critical role of your genetics in determining your nutritional requirements, how to decode your DNA for personalized nutrition, and the importance of working with a qualified healthcare professional to create a diet plan tailored to your genetic blueprint.

3.1.1 Nutrigenomics: The science of nutrition and genetics

Nutrigenomics is the study of the intersection between human genomics, nutrition, and health. It seeks to understand how our genetic variations influence our response to nutrients and how this response can affect our well-being. The goal of nutrigenomics is to provide personalized dietary recommendations, based on your unique genetic code, to prevent, mitigate, or treat certain diseases, conditions, and to improve overall health.

One key aspect of nutrigenomics is understanding how genetic variants called single nucleotide polymorphisms (SNPs) can affect our metabolism and response to dietary components. These SNPs can alter the way our body processes certain nutrients, leading to different health outcomes and a need for personalized nutrition.

3.1.2 Identifying critical SNPs for personalized nutrition

Every person carries numerous SNPs that influence their response to food and nutrients. Some well-known examples include:

1. **MTHFR gene:** This gene is involved in the metabolism of folate and vitamin B12, essential nutrients for DNA synthesis and repair. Variants in this gene can result in reduced efficiency of folate metabolism, potentially leading to elevated levels of homocysteine, which has been linked to an increased risk of cardiovascular disease and other health issues. Personalized nutrition for individuals with these variants may include supplementation with the more active form of folate, called methylfolate.
2. **APOE gene:** The APOE gene is responsible for producing a protein that transports cholesterol and other fats throughout the body. Variants in this gene can impact cholesterol levels and cardiovascular health. People carrying the APOE ε4 variant have an increased risk of developing heart disease and Alzheimer's disease. Personalized diet recommendations for ε4 carriers may include emphasizing mono- and polyunsaturated fats while minimizing saturated and trans fats.
3. **LCT gene:** The LCT gene is responsible for producing lactase, the enzyme that breaks down

lactose, a sugar found in milk and dairy products. Some individuals carry an SNP in this gene that leads to lactose intolerance, characterized by gas, bloating, and other digestive symptoms after consuming dairy. Personalized dietary strategies for lactose intolerant individuals could include avoiding or limiting dairy, or using lactase supplements to aid digestion.

3.1.3 Putting it all together: Personalizing your diet based on your genetics

Once we have identified critical SNPs and the genetic variations that cause altered metabolism, we can create personalized dietary recommendations to optimize your nutritional intake. Here are some general pointers for personalizing your diet based on your genetic makeup:

1. **Consult a professional:** Work with a registered dietitian or certified nutrition specialist who is experienced in genomics and personalized nutrition. They can help you interpret your genetic data and create a customized diet plan to address your specific nutritional needs.
2. **Prioritize whole, unprocessed foods:** Regardless of your genetics, a diet rich in whole, unprocessed plant and animal foods provides a variety of essential nutrients needed for good health.
3. **Personalize your macronutrient ratios:** Depending on your genetic predisposition, you may have a higher need for carbohydrates, fats, or proteins in your diet. A personalized macronutrient ratio can help you achieve optimal energy levels, body composition, and overall health.
4. **Address micronutrient needs:** Depending on your genetic makeup, you may have unique requirements for specific vitamins and minerals. A personalized diet

plan can help ensure you consume sufficient amounts of these micronutrients to support your genetic potential.

5. **Consider personalized supplementation:** If you are unable to get all the necessary nutrients from your diet or have specific genetic requirements, targeted supplementation might be beneficial. Only add supplements under the supervision of a qualified healthcare professional.

3.1.4 In conclusion

Our genetic makeup plays a significant role in determining our nutritional needs and how we respond to certain foods. Unlocking the potential of personalized nutrition through the understanding of nutrigenomics is an exciting and evolving field that can contribute significantly to our health and well-being. By adopting a personalized diet based on your unique genetic blueprint, you can lay the foundation for optimal health and longevity.

The Importance of Genetic Profiling for a Biohacker's Diet

A crucial aspect of the biohacker's quest for optimal health lies in the domain of personal nutrition. By deciphering your genetic blueprints, you can strategize your dietary choices to work in harmony with your body, achieving an equilibrium that not only enhances your physical and mental performance but also secures long-term wellness. This section will delve into the realm of genetic profiling, providing the tools and knowledge necessary to construct a personalized diet that serves as the foundation for exceptional health.

Unraveling the Genetic Code: Demystifying DNA

In order to design a nutrition plan tailored to your genes, it is essential to first understand the underlying principles of genetics. At its core, deoxyribonucleic acid (DNA) comprises a sequence of building blocks known as nucleotides. These nucleotides come together to form units called genes, which serve as the blueprints for proteins—the workhorses of the cell responsible for carrying out a wide array of functions, from breaking down nutrients to combating infections.

Crucially, variations within genes can radically impact how individuals respond to different types of nutrients. By analyzing these genetic variations, it is possible to identify the optimal balance of macronutrients (fats, proteins, and carbohydrates) and micronutrients (vitamins and minerals) to ensure that your body functions at peak capacity.

Decoding the Nutrigenomic Landscape: Identifying Your Nutritional Archetypes

Nutrigenomics, the study of how nutrients interact with our genes, has come to the forefront of dietary research in recent years. By assessing specific genes linked to nutrient metabolism, scientists can now delineate an individual's unique nutritional needs, breaking down genetic data into distinct "archetypes."

These archetypes include, but are not limited to:

1. *Carbohydrate Metabolism*: Determines how efficiently your body breaks down carbohydrates, impacting energy levels and weight management.
2. *Fat Metabolism*: Dictates how effectively your body is able to break down and utilize fats, influencing weight, inflammation, and cardiovascular health.

3. *Protein Metabolism*: Reveals how well your body processes proteins, affecting muscle growth, recovery, and metabolic rate.
4. *Micronutrient Needs*: Identifies specific vitamin and mineral requirements, ensuring cellular health and preventing deficiencies.
5. *Food Sensitivities*: Uncovers possible intolerances to various nutrients, such as lactose, gluten, or caffeine.

By comprehending these archetypes, you can optimize your diet to fuel your body's unique genetic composition.

Combining the Data: Creating Your Personalized Nutrition Plan

Once you have a clear understanding of your genetic profile, the next step is synthesizing the information to create a diet tailored to your specific needs. Here are some key considerations when designing your personalized nutrition plan:

1. *Macronutrient Ratios*: Depending on your genetic predispositions, adjust your fat, protein, and carbohydrate ratios to align with your metabolic needs. For instance, individuals with a genetic propensity for carbohydrate sensitivity may need to adopt a low-carbohydrate, high-fat diet to support weight management and satiety.
2. *Food Selection*: Choose foods that align with your genetic profile. For example, if your genes indicate a higher need for omega-3 fatty acids, incorporate fatty fish, walnuts, or flax seeds into your diet.
3. *Supplementation*: To supplement for any micronutrient deficiencies your genetic profile may reveal, consider integrating high-quality vitamins, minerals, and other nutrients into your daily routine.

4. *Mindful Eating*: Cultivating a mindful approach to food can help you attune to your body's unique hunger and satiety signals, supporting weight management and overall health.
5. *Adjustments*: Continuously monitor your body's response to your personalized diet and make adjustments as needed to ensure optimal results.

A Lifetime of Nutritional Mastery: The Biohacker's Commitment

By embarking on this journey toward nutritional mastery, you are taking an essential step toward forging not only improved physical health but also a more intimate connection with your body's ultimate design. Through ongoing refinement and commitment to your personalized diet, you can elevate your well-being and establish a foundation for a lifetime of vitality and wellness. Your genetic destiny awaits.

3.1 Understanding Your Unique Genetic Makeup

Before diving into the world of biohacking and tailoring your diet to suit your specific genetic needs, it's essential to first understand how genetics play a role in determining our body's response to food and exercise. Our genes are the blueprint for our body's functions and are passed down from our parents. Some of the traits that we commonly associate with genetics, such as hair color and height, can also be reflected in various metabolic processes, nutrient absorption and even food preferences.

a) Nutrigenomics - The "Nature" Aspect of Diet

Nutrigenomics is a relatively new field that studies how our genes interact with the nutrients we consume, and how it affects our overall health. It's the science behind the concept that certain foods might be more beneficial for some individuals, while others may not reap the same rewards from consuming the same food. The idea is based on the understanding that our genes are capable of influencing our body's ability to absorb, utilize, and store nutrients. Knowing your genetic makeup can provide a deeper insight into how your body processes certain nutrients, and help you make informed decisions about what to eat.

For example, some people have a genetic predisposition to digest lactose, the sugar found in dairy products, while others may have difficulty processing it. This is primarily due to a genetic variation in the LCT gene that determines the level of lactase (the enzyme responsible for breaking down lactose) in the body. By understanding this genetic factor, an individual with lactose intolerance can choose alternative, lactose-free sources of calcium to better suit their genetic needs, such as almond or soy milk, fortified orange juice or kale.

b) Epigenetics - The "Nurture" Factor in Diet

While our genes play a role in determining our optimal diet, our environment and lifestyle choices can influence how those genes are expressed or "switched on." Epigenetics, the study of modifications in our gene expression, reveals that the expression of certain genes can be altered by external factors, such as stress, exposure to toxins, and – you guessed it – diet.

For years, food has been considered more than just a source of nutrients; it can be considered as a signal that can affect gene expression. An unhealthy diet can negatively impact genes associated with metabolism, which in turn can lead to complications like obesity or type 2 diabetes. By understanding the impact of our dietary choices on our genetic expression, we can make better decisions to optimize our health and well-being.

c) Identifying Your Genetic Profile

To start personalizing your diet according to your genetic makeup, the first step is to understand your genetic profile. This can be done with the help of direct-to-consumer genetic testing services like 23andMe, AncestryDNA, or Nutrigenomix. These platforms can provide you with a detailed report of your genetic variants, their associated health implications, and how they relate to your nutrient requirements or food sensitivities.

For instance, a genetic report may reveal that you have a higher likelihood of developing type 2 diabetes. In this case, it would be essential to prioritize a more significant proportion of low-glycemic foods, such as whole grains and legumes, in your diet to keep blood sugar levels under control. Alternatively, some individuals may have variations in genes related to fat metabolism, suggesting they might benefit from consuming a diet higher in monounsaturated and polyunsaturated fats while minimizing saturated fat consumption to maintain optimal health.

3.1.1 Crafting Your Personalized Diet Plan

Now that you have a better understanding of how genetics and epigenetics influence your dietary requirements and preferences, it's time to put that knowledge to work. The following steps will guide you in creating the perfect diet plan tailored to your unique genetic makeup:

1. **Prioritize nutrient-rich foods:** No matter your genetic profile, it is always essential to consume a nutrient-dense diet, including whole foods like fruits, vegetables, whole grains, lean proteins, and healthy fats. These foods will not only provide the nutrients and energy needed for optimal health, but they can also have a positive effect on gene expression.

2. **Optimize macro and micronutrient ratios:** Based on your genetic profile, you may have varying requirements for specific macronutrients (carbohydrates, fats, and proteins) or micronutrients (vitamins and minerals). Aim to strike a balance that matches your genetic needs as closely as possible, keeping in mind that these ratios may change with time as your activity levels, health goals, or life stage changes.

3. **Address food sensitivities or allergies:** Your genetic test results may reveal certain food sensitivities or allergies to specific dietary components, such as lactose or gluten. Listen to your body and adjust your diet to avoid such triggers or find suitable alternatives to ensure you maintain optimal health.

4. **Listen to your body:** As you implement your personalized diet plan, monitor how you feel physically and mentally. Your body is unique, and it might take some trial and error to find the optimal nutrition plan. Pay attention to your energy levels, digestion, mood, and any changes in your physique – these signs will tell you if your diet is on the right track or if you need to make additional adjustments.

5. **Reassess and evolve:** Remember that our bodies change over time, and what worked for you once might not necessarily work forever. Regularly reevaluating your diet plan and making adjustments to accommodate shifts in lifestyle or health status will

ensure that you continue to thrive and maintain optimal wellbeing.

In conclusion, personalizing your diet according to your genetic makeup and understanding the role of both nature and nurture in shaping your nutritional requirements can serve as a foundation for optimal health. By taking the steps outlined in this section, you can create a customized nutrition plan that addresses your unique needs, empowers your genetic potential, and sets you up for long-term success.

3.1 Uncovering Your Genetic Tendencies

Before diving into personalized diet recommendations designed for genetic success, it's important to gain an understanding of how our genes influence our nutritional needs and preferences. Your DNA is unique, and so too are your natural tendencies and predispositions towards certain types of foods and nutrients that can help or hinder your journey toward optimal health.

A. Understanding Your Genetic Makeup

Your genetic makeup is the culmination of your inherited traits passed down from your ancestors. These traits not only include the way you look but also influence how your body functions on a cellular level. Genes, the working units of heredity, contribute to your individual needs for specific nutrients and have an impact on how your body processes and utilizes these nutrients.

Example: *APOE gene*

A widely studied gene, APOE, is associated with the risk of developing Alzheimer's disease. This gene exists in three different forms: APOE2, APOE3, and APOE4. Individuals carrying the APOE4 variant have an increased risk of Alzheimer's by up to 12 times, compared to those without this variant. As a result, specific dietary recommendations can help those with the APOE4 variant to reduce their risk of cognitive decline.

By understanding your genetic makeup, you can create a tailored diet that complements your inherited traits and maximizes your potential for optimal health.

B. Genetic Testing: The Key to Personalized Nutrition

To begin unlocking the power of your genes and creating a personalized diet plan, genetic testing is a great starting point. These tests involve analyzing your DNA, typically through a saliva sample, and can provide you with a wealth of information on your unique genetic variations. Genetic testing companies, such as 23andMe, AncestryDNA, and Nutrigenomix, offer a range of testing services, from ancestry to specific health and wellness-focused tests.

The results of these tests can help you identify specific areas of your diet that may require adjustment based on your genetic predispositions. For example, some people may require more or less of certain nutrients, like vitamin D or omega-3 fatty acids, based on their individual genetic blueprint.

Once you've received your genetic results, it's essential to work with a healthcare professional or nutritionist to interpret the data and apply it to your dietary plan.

C. Harnessing the Power of Nutrigenomics

Nutrigenomics is the study of how our genes interact with the nutrients we consume. By understanding the relationship between our genes and the foods we eat, we can design an optimal diet tailored to our unique genetic makeup. This revolutionary field of study reinforces the notion that one-size-fits-all dietary advice may not be applicable to everyone.

As you uncover your genetic tendencies through testing, it's essential to consider the following factors when making dietary decisions:

1. **Nutrient requirements**: Your body may require more or less of certain nutrients, such as vitamins, minerals, amino acids, or fatty acids, based on your genetic makeup.
2. **Food sensitivities and intolerances**: Some individuals have genetic predispositions to adverse reactions from specific foods or food components, such as lactose, gluten, or histamine.
3. **Energy balance and metabolism**: Your genes can influence how efficiently your body uses energy from food and how it stores or burns fat.
4. **Appetite regulation**: Several genetic factors can affect your appetite, satiety, and food craving behaviors.
5. **Taste preference**: Genetic differences can also impact your taste preferences, making certain foods more appealing or less palatable to you.

By considering these factors, you'll be better equipped to create a personalized diet plan that is designed specifically for your genetic success.

D. Creating Your Personalized Diet Plan

Once you've discovered your unique genetic tendencies, it's time to put the knowledge into action by tailoring your diet to cater to your individual needs.

1. **Consult with a professional**: A registered dietitian or nutritionist trained in nutrigenomics can help you translate your genetic information into practical and actionable dietary recommendations.
2. **Adjust macronutrient ratios**: Depending on your genetic makeup, you may benefit from consuming more or fewer carbohydrates, proteins, or fats. Adjusting these ratios can optimize your energy levels and metabolism based on your genetic predispositions.
3. **Prioritize micronutrients**: Incorporate foods rich in specific vitamins, minerals, and other nutrients that your body particularly requires or processes efficiently, as determined by your genetic results.
4. **Address food sensitivities**: If your test results show that you may be predisposed to intolerances or sensitivities to certain foods or components, consider eliminating these from your diet or reducing their intake to avoid potential adverse effects on your health.
5. **Monitor and adjust**: Regularly evaluate your progress and, if necessary, adjust your dietary plan. Your needs may change over time, and staying in tune with your body will help you maintain optimal health through personalized nutrition.

By personalizing your diet based on your unique genetic blueprint, you can maximize your potential for achieving and maintaining optimal health. Remember that an optimal diet is about more than just weight loss or maintenance - it's about fueling your body to achieve its fullest potential in all aspects of health and performance. With the insights provided by genetic testing and a carefully designed diet plan, you'll be well on your way toward mastering your nutrition and unlocking your ultimate health potential.

Genetic Variation: One Size Doesn't Fit All

The first step to Personalizing Your Diet for Genetic Success is understanding that everyone's bodies have unique genetic variation. This genetic variation, known as single nucleotide polymorphisms (SNPs), are small differences in the DNA sequence that can result in altered protein production, leading to diverse physiological responses to the same stimulus. Consequently, the way you respond to particular foods can be quite different from the way your friend or family member would.

Nutrigenomics: Bridging the Gap between Genetics and Nutrition

Nutrigenomics is the scientific discipline that investigates the interaction between the foods we consume and our genetic makeup. By understanding this relationship, a personalized diet can be devised that takes into account the genetic predispositions of each individual.

The primary objective of nutrigenomics is to identify the specific nutrients and bioactive compounds in foods that help or harm us based on our unique genetic variation, allowing for the tailoring of dietary recommendations to support optimal health.

Common Genetic Variations that Impact Nutrition

There are numerous genetic variations that can have an impact on how we respond to certain foods, particularly regarding macronutrient metabolism, food sensitivities, and micronutrient requirements. Some common examples include:

1. **APOE gene variations**: The APOE gene is involved in cholesterol transport and metabolism. Some variations of this gene, particularly APOE4, is associated with a higher risk of heart disease and Alzheimer's disease. Individuals with the APOE4 allele may benefit from a lower fat diet, particularly when it comes to saturated fats.
2. **MTHFR gene variations**: The MTHFR gene regulates the conversion of folate, a B-vitamin, into its active form known as methylfolate. MTHFR gene variations can decrease the efficiency of this conversion process, increasing the risk for a higher level of homocysteine, which is linked to heart disease and other health issues. Individuals with this genetic variation may benefit from additional folate in their diet or supplementation with methylfolate.
3. **CYP1A2 gene variations**: This gene influences the rate at which the body metabolizes caffeine. Some variations result in slower caffeine metabolism, while others lead to faster metabolism. Slow metabolizers are at greater risk for heart disease when consuming a high-caffeine diet over an extended period.
4. **Gluten sensitivity and Celiac disease**: Several genes have been associated with an increased risk of

developing Celiac disease, a severe autoimmune condition triggered by the ingestion of gluten. Some individuals without Celiac disease are also susceptible to gluten sensitivity, leading to digestive issues and other symptoms. Genetic testing can reveal whether implementing a gluten-free diet would be beneficial based on the presence of specific genes.

5. **Lactose intolerance**: A genetic variation in the LCT gene can lead to lactose intolerance, a condition in which the body cannot break down lactose, a sugar found in milk and milk-based products, causing digestive discomfort. Adjusting the diet to include lactose-free options can alleviate symptoms in these individuals.

How to Personalize Your Diet for Genetic Success

As our understanding of the relationship between genetics and nutrition evolves, it becomes increasingly clear that adhering to a one-size-fits-all approach is an oversimplification of the complex ways our bodies interact with food.

To begin incorporating the principles of nutrigenomics into your life:

1. **Get tested**: Several genetic testing services available today can offer insights into your unique genetic makeup, including genotyping of various genes related to nutrition.
2. **Work with a professional**: Consult with a nutrition professional, such as a registered dietitian, who is experienced in nutrigenomics. They can help you interpret your genetic data and offer personalized recommendations.

3. **Adjust your diet**: Based on the findings from genetic testing, work with your healthcare provider to create a customized meal plan that accounts for the unique genetic factors influencing your nutritional needs.
4. **Monitor and adapt**: Track your progress over time, noting any improvements or setbacks in your health. As with any diet, adjusting your intake of specific nutrients, food groups, and macronutrients may be necessary as your body evolves and your nutritional needs change.

By considering your unique genetic makeup when designing your diet, you can move toward a more personalized and effective approach to better health.

4. Fitness Optimization: Tailoring Training Programs for Your Unique Body

4.1 Individualizing Nutrition to Fuel Your Training

Nutrition is a crucial, non-negotiable component of any fitness program. Biohacking requires a personalized approach to nutrition, recognizing that each person's dietary needs are unique. Tailoring a nutrition plan to the individual's specific needs, preferences, and goals will ultimately lead to better training outcomes and overall health. The following steps provide a blueprint to optimize your nutrition, fuel your workouts and deliver maximum results:

1. Determine your energy needs

Understanding the caloric intake required to maintain, lose or gain weight is the first step in creating a customized nutrition plan. Use an online calculator or work with a dietician to determine your basal metabolic rate (BMR) – the energy your body requires to maintain normal functioning at rest. Then, factor in your activity level to calculate your total energy expenditure (TDEE). This will give you a starting point to modify caloric intake depending on your goals – weight loss, weight maintenance, or bulking.

2. Analyze your macronutrient ratios

Macronutrients – protein, fat, and carbohydrates – are the major components of our diet, each serving specific functions. Protein supports muscle growth and repair, fat supports hormonal and brain health, and carbohydrates fuel high-intensity exercise. Determining the right nutrient ratios involves establishing the proper balance of these macronutrients for your individual needs. General guidelines are:

- Protein: 1.4g - 2g per kilogram of body weight per day
- Fat: 0.7g - 1g per kilogram of body weight per day
- Carbohydrates: The remaining caloric intake after protein and fat requirements are met

Use these recommendations as a starting point, listening to your body and adjusting as necessary. A registered dietician or advanced biohacker apps can also provide valuable guidance.

3. Optimize nutrient timing

Nutrient timing refers to the strategic intake of specific nutrients around your training sessions to maximize the benefits of your workouts. Consuming an appropriate balance of carbs and protein pre- and post- workout can support recovery, muscle growth, and performance. Common guidelines include:

- Pre-workout snack (1-2 hours before training): Focus on a mix of carbohydrates and protein to fuel your workout and minimize muscle breakdown. Aim for a 3:1 carb to protein ratio.
- Post-workout nourishment (within 30-60 minutes after training): Prioritize recovery with a meal or snack containing both carbohydrates and protein, with a 31 or 41 carb to protein ratio. This combination helps replenish glycogen levels and facilitate muscle repair.

4. Prioritize quality and nutrient density

Eating high-quality, nutrient-dense foods is fundamental to fueling your body effectively. Consuming a variety of colorful fruits and vegetables, whole grains, lean proteins, and healthy fats will provide energy, promote muscle growth, and reduce inflammation. Pay attention to the quality of your food sources, opting for organic produce, grass-fed meats, and wild-caught fish when possible.

5. Investigate food sensitivities

Undiagnosed or unrecognized food sensitivities may contribute to gut dysfunction, inflammation, and impaired recovery. An elimination or low-FODMAP diet can be helpful in identifying trigger foods, allowing you to create a personalized diet that supports gut health and reduces inflammation. Consult a registered dietician for guidance on implementing these diets.

6. Monitor, adjust, and adapt

The human body is a complex, adaptive system, constantly evolving and responding to external stimuli. To optimize your nutritional strategy, closely monitor your body's response to your dietary choices. Maintain a detailed food journal, noting your energy levels, mood, sleep quality, digestive health, and physical performance. Regularly re-evaluate and adjust your nutrition plan as needed, celebrating progress and remaining open to change.

In summary, an individualized approach to nutrition is essential to optimize health and training performance. By understanding your energy needs, macronutrient ratios, nutrient timing, and appropriate food choices, you will be better equipped to fuel your body effectively, maximize results, and biohack your way to optimal health.

4.1 Understanding Your Body Type and Genetic Predispositions: The Key to Personalized Fitness

No two people have the exact same body. Just as we all have our unique fingerprints, we also have our unique body types, genetic predispositions, and fitness goals. To optimize your fitness and health, it is crucial to understand the nuances of your own body and create a training program that is tailored specifically to your needs. In this section, we will explore the different aspects of your body that will help determine the most effective and efficient training program to help you reach your goals.

A. Assessing Your Body Type: Ectomorph, Mesomorph, or Endomorph?

When it comes to body types, there are three primary categories: ectomorphs, mesomorphs, and endomorphs.

Your body type plays a significant role in determining how you should approach your fitness routine. Although people often have a combination of these body types, identifying your dominant body type can help fine-tune your training approach.

1. **Ectomorphs** are characterized by a lean, slender frame with a fast metabolism. They generally have difficulty gaining weight, both muscle mass and fat. Ectomorphs often have a hard time building muscle and need to focus on strength training and eating a calorie surplus to achieve muscle growth. They may also benefit from shorter, more intense workouts to avoid burning too many calories.
2. **Mesomorphs** have a naturally athletic build with a balanced musculoskeletal structure. They are naturally strong and can gain muscle mass relatively easily. Due to their natural propensity for athleticism, they can benefit from a variety of training methods, focusing on both strength and endurance. Mesomorphs should strive for a well-rounded fitness routine that incorporates a balance of strength training, cardiovascular exercises, and flexibility training.
3. **Endomorphs** have a larger frame and tend to carry more body fat than the other types. They may struggle with weight loss and fat accumulation, especially around the midsection. Endomorphs should focus on cardiovascular exercises to help burn fat and promote weight loss. While strength training is still important, it should be combined with a regular cardio routine and a calorie-controlled diet to help shed excess body fat.

Knowing your body type can help you tailor your training program to better suit your individual needs and goals. By focusing on your unique strengths and weaknesses, you can optimize your workout routine to achieve the results you desire.

B. Evaluating Your Genetic Predispositions

In addition to your body type, your genetic predispositions can also influence your training and fitness goals. Certain genetic factors can impact your muscle fiber makeup, cardiovascular fitness, and overall athletic ability. By understanding your genetic predispositions, you can tailor your training program to focus on areas that require more attention.

1. **Muscle Fiber Makeup**: Your muscles are composed of a combination of slow-twitch and fast-twitch fibers. Slow-twitch fibers are more efficient at using oxygen and are suited for endurance activities, while fast-twitch fibers are better for short bursts of power and strength. Your genetic makeup plays a role in the proportion of these fibers in your muscles. By focusing your training on your dominant muscle fiber type (i.e., emphasizing endurance exercises for slow-twitch dominant individuals), you can maximize your athletic potential.
2. **Cardiovascular Fitness**: Genetics also play a role in your aerobic capacity, or how efficiently your body can use oxygen during exercise. Those with a higher genetic predisposition for cardiovascular fitness will naturally be able to perform better in aerobic activities such as running or swimming. Tailoring your training to capitalize on this strength can help optimize your workout routine.
3. **Athletic Ability**: Some individuals are naturally more predisposed to excel in athletic activities. While it is important to recognize that genetics can only take you so far, understanding your natural abilities can help

guide your training program. Focusing on activities that align with your genetic predispositions can lead to greater enjoyment and success in your fitness journey.

C. Setting Your Fitness Goals: The SMART Approach

To help tailor your training program to your unique body, it is essential to set clear, specific fitness goals. One popular method for goal-setting is the SMART approach, which stands for Specific, Measurable, Achievable, Relevant, and Time-bound.

1. **Specific**: Your goals should be clearly defined and easy to understand. Instead of setting a vague goal like "I want to get in shape", aim for a specific objective, such as "I want to lose 10 pounds" or "I want to run a half-marathon in under two hours".
2. **Measurable**: Ensure your goals can be measured so that you can track your progress. For instance, if your goal is to build muscle, track your increases in weight lifted or changes in muscle circumference.
3. **Achievable**: Set realistic goals that are both challenging and attainable. Consider your current fitness level, time constraints, and available resources when establishing your objectives.
4. **Relevant**: Your goals should align with your personal interests, values, and long-term objectives. This ensures that you are motivated and committed to achieving your goals, leading to a higher likelihood of success.
5. **Time-bound**: Establish a timeframe for achieving your goals, whether that be weeks, months, or years. This helps create a sense of urgency and motivation towards your objectives.

By setting SMART goals, you can tailor your training program to focus on the specific tasks and activities that will lead to the achievement of your unique fitness objectives.

D. Putting It All Together: Creating Your Personalized Training Program

With an understanding of your body type, genetic predispositions, and personal fitness goals, you can now begin to create a personalized training program. This program should focus on exercises and activities that will help achieve your specific objectives while capitalizing on your unique strengths and addressing your particular weaknesses. Consider incorporating the following elements when designing your training program:

1. **Exercise Selection**: Choose exercises that align with your goals and cater to your body type and genetic predispositions. For instance, an ectomorph looking to build muscle should focus on compound strength training exercises, while an endomorph aiming for weight loss should prioritize cardiovascular exercises.
2. **Intensity and Volume**: The intensity and volume of your workouts should be tailored to your current fitness level and desired results. Gradually increase these variables over time as your body adapts and your fitness improves.
3. **Frequency**: Determine how often you will exercise based on your goals, body type, and lifestyle. Ensure that your training frequency allows for adequate recovery time and prevents overtraining or burnout.
4. **Progressions**: To prevent plateaus and ensure continued progress towards your goals, incorporate progressions into your training routine. This can include increasing the intensity, volume, or frequency

of your workouts, or altering the exercises and activities themselves.

5. **Rest and Recovery**: Recognize the importance of rest and recovery in achieving your fitness goals. Schedule regular rest days and ensure proper sleep, nutrition, and stress management to support your training program.

By considering these factors and building a training routine tailored to your unique body and objectives, you can optimize your fitness journey and achieve the results you desire. Embrace your individuality and take control of your health with a fitness program designed specifically for you.

4.1 Understanding Your Genetic Fingerprint: Tracking the Right Metrics

Understanding your genetic makeup is a crucial factor in tailoring your training program for optimal fitness. This subset of biohacking utilizes DNA analysis to identify your specific body type and the most effective exercise strategies for you. To truly unlock your physical potential, you must first learn which genes make up your unique genetic fingerprint.

A. The Role of Genetics in Fitness

Your genetic makeup determines a broad spectrum of traits, including athleticism, susceptibility to certain health conditions, and even personal preferences. As recent technological advancements have made genomic testing more accessible, it has become easier than ever to take a deep dive into your genes in order to maximize your fitness success. One way to gather information for your optimal health blueprint is through direct-to-consumer genetic testing offered by companies like 23andMe, Ancestry, or MyHeritage. By analyzing your genetic data, these companies provide personalized insights into your overall health, disease risk, and traits connected to athletic performance.

B. Genetic Testing for Fitness Optimization

As you begin to explore the world of genetic testing, it's important to recognize four major gene categories that play a key role in fitness optimization:

1. **Body Composition & Muscle Fiber:** By analyzing genes like ACTN3, ACVR2B, or MSTN, a genetic test can offer insight into your body's natural lean mass distribution or the type of muscle fibers that dominate, which can help identify the optimal workout strategies for your body.
2. **Cardiorespiratory Fitness & Endurance:** Certain genes such as ACE, ADRB2 or PPARA have an impact on your body's cardiovascular response to training, arterial flexibility, and even the ability to produce aerobic energy. This information can help determine whether you may fare better focusing on endurance-based workouts or predominantly aerobic activities, such as swimming or cycling.
3. **Inflammation & Injury Risk:** Genes like IL6 or COL1A1 give insight into how efficiently your body handles inflammation as well as its natural susceptibility to joint and tendon injuries. Being aware of this data can help you tailor workouts, recovery strategies, and supplementary regimens to minimize injury risk and maximize recovery efficiency.
4. **Nutrient Metabolism:** Lastly, genes like FTO, MC4R, or CYP1A2 provide information on how your body processes vitamins, minerals, and other key nutrients,

which can inform custom nutritional plans based on your genetic profile.

C. Tracking Your Fitness Metrics

Once you've gathered information through genetic testing, it's essential to track the right metrics for your specific genetic profile. Establishing this personalized performance dashboard equips you with information necessary to make informed changes to your training regimen, nutrition plan, and overall lifestyle. Common fitness metrics include:

1. **Resting Heart Rate (RHR):** A good indicator of your overall cardiovascular health, which is influenced by genes like ACE and ADRB2. Tracking your RHR over time allows you to evaluate your aerobic capacity and the effectiveness of your endurance-based workouts.
2. **VO2 Max:** This metric measures the maximum amount of oxygen your body can utilize during intense activity, which is directly influenced by genes such as PPARA and NRF2. Keeping tabs on your VO2 max can help you assess your cardiovascular fitness and the potential improvements gained from your tailored exercise plan.
3. **Strength & Power Measurements:** By tracking muscular strength and power through one-rep max lifts, sprint times, or vertical jump tests, you can gauge the efficacy of your personalized strength-training plan based on your body composition and muscle fiber type.
4. **Body Composition Metrics:** Tracking body fat percentage, lean muscle mass, and other body composition metrics allows you to monitor changes in your overall physique over time in relation to your specific genetic makeup.

5. **Injury & Recovery Assessments:** Pay close attention to signs of inflammation, injury-related pain, or slow recovery as you track your progress. Address these issues with appropriate measures, such as adjusting workout intensity or implementing additional recovery methods like stretching, massage, or ice therapy.

D. Adapting Your Training Program

With your genetic fingerprint in hand and powerful metrics tracked over time, you can modify your program to capitalize on strengths, address weaknesses, and ultimately develop a powerful, efficient body. Don't be afraid to shift your focus, switch up routines, or fine-tune your diet to match your genetic predispositions.

In the quest for optimized health and fitness, understanding your unique genetic fingerprint is critical. Genetic testing, tailored training programs, and diligent tracking of the right metrics will lead you to the fullest expression of your physical potential. Always remember that the path to optimal health is a journey of self-discovery, exploration, and continuous adaptation. Stay curious and remain open to the transformative potential of new data as you sculpt your body by design.

4.1 Understanding Your Body Type: The First Step To A Tailored Training Program

Before diving into the world of fitness optimization, it's crucial to understand your body type, as this will significantly influence the types of workouts and nutrition that will work best for you in your journey towards optimal health. There are three primary body types, known as somatotypes:

1. **Ectomorph:** Characterized by a lean, slim build, ectomorphs usually have narrow shoulders, fast metabolism, and smaller muscles. People with this body type often have difficulties gaining weight and muscle mass.
2. **Mesomorph:** This body type is characterized by an athletic, muscular build with broad shoulders, developed muscles, and a strong metabolism. They can typically gain and lose weight relatively easily.
3. **Endomorph:** Endomorphs typically have a bigger, rounder build, with wider hips and shoulders, slower metabolism, and a greater propensity to store fat. They may find it more challenging to lose weight and keep it off.

Understanding your somatotype will help to guide you in developing a training program that caters to your body type and goals. In this section, we'll outline how each somatotype can approach fitness optimization for the best results.

4.1.1 Tailoring Training For Ectomorphs

Since ectomorphs have a leaner physique, a main goal may be to gain muscle mass and increase strength. To achieve this, ectomorphs should:

1. **Focus on compound weightlifting exercises** such as squats, deadlifts, bench press, and rows. These exercises work multiple muscle groups simultaneously and allow for heavier weights, promoting optimal muscle growth.
2. **Limit cardiovascular training** to avoid burning excessive calories needed for muscle growth. Low-

intensity, steady-state cardio (like brisk walking) can be beneficial for overall health without hindering mass gains.

3. **Prioritize rest and recovery** to promote muscle growth. Aim for 7-9 hours of sleep each night and schedule rest days between intense lifting sessions to allow the body time to rebuild and grow.
4. **Consume adequate calories and macronutrients** to support muscle growth. Ectomorphs should focus on eating a surplus of high-quality calories to fuel their workouts and increase muscle mass, ensuring that they consume sufficient amounts of protein, carbohydrates, and healthy fats.

4.1.2 Tailoring Training For Mesomorphs

Given their naturally athletic and muscular physique, mesomorphs can adapt to varying training styles. Some key points for mesomorphs to consider:

1. **Incorporate a mix of strength and endurance training** to maintain and build muscle mass while staying lean. This can include a combination of weightlifting, bodyweight exercises, and cardiovascular workouts.
2. **Experiment with workout intensity and volume** to find the right balance for your goals. Mesomorphs can benefit from high-intensity training, but must be mindful of overtraining, which can lead to injuries or excessive muscle loss.
3. **Track your progress and make adjustments** as needed. Mesomorphs have the unique ability to gain and lose weight more easily, so regularly monitoring progress can help fine-tune training and nutrition to continue moving towards your goals.

4. **Eat a balanced, nutrient-dense diet** to fuel workouts and maintain a lean physique. Mesomorphs should ensure they consume enough protein to support muscle growth while also getting adequate carbohydrates for energy and healthy fats for hormonal balance and overall health.

4.1.3 Tailoring Training For Endomorphs

Given their propensity to store fat, endomorphs may find it challenging to lose weight and maintain a lean physique. To overcome this challenge, endomorphs should:

1. **Prioritize cardiovascular training** to increase caloric expenditure and promote fat loss. Incorporate both steady-state and high-intensity interval training (HIIT) for optimal results.
2. **Include muscle-building exercises** like weightlifting and bodyweight movements to increase muscle mass and further support fat loss attempts. By building more muscle, endomorphs can improve their metabolic rate and burn more calories at rest.
3. **Monitor nutrition closely** to ensure a calorie deficit is achieved while still providing adequate nutrients for health and energy. Focus on a high-protein, moderate-carb, and low-fat diet to support both weight loss and muscle retention.
4. **Implement stress reduction and sleep optimization techniques** as high stress levels and poor sleep can negatively impact endomorphs' ability to lose weight. Aim for 7-9 hours of quality sleep per night and practice stress-management techniques like meditation, deep breathing, or engaging in relaxing hobbies.

By understanding your body type and tailoring your training program accordingly, you'll be well on your way to achieving optimal fitness and health. Remember, patience, consistency, and perseverance are key, as results may not happen overnight. Keep refining your personalized fitness blueprint as you progress, and enjoy the journey towards a healthier and fitter version of yourself.

Customizing Workouts: The Key to Unlocking Your Fitness Potential

Every individual is unique, and hence, a one-size-fits-all approach to fitness is rarely as effective as a personalized and targeted training program. Optimizing your fitness routine according to your unique body type, goals, and abilities will not only help you achieve your desired outcome faster, but it will also make the process more enjoyable and sustainable. In this subsection, we'll explore essential factors to consider while crafting a custom-tailored workout plan, ensuring that you're functioning at your peak and catering to your body's specific needs.

Understanding Your Body Type

Before customizing your workout plan, you need to understand your body type or somatotype. There are usually three body types - ectomorph, mesomorph, and endomorph. Ectomorphs are generally characterized by their lean and thin stature, making it challenging to gain both muscle and fat. Mesomorphs are individuals with a muscular build, making it easier for them to gain muscle and lose fat. Endomorphs tend to have a higher body fat percentage, and while they can gain muscle easily, losing fat can be challenging.

Being aware of your body type enables you to adjust your workout routine, ensuring that you're focusing on the appropriate exercises and training styles. It is vital to remember that body types do not exist in isolation, and most people display a mixture of somatotypes, so it's essential to consider your individual characteristics.

Determine Your Fitness Goals

Setting clear and measurable goals is crucial for creating a tailored workout plan that addresses your specific needs. Whether your goal is weight loss, muscle gain, increasing flexibility, or improving cardiovascular endurance, defining these objectives will influence the type of exercises and training styles to focus on. Additionally, it's beneficial to establish short- and long-term goals, promoting a sense of motivation and allowing for progressive improvements over time.

Incorporate the Right Training Styles

Depending on your body type and fitness goals, different training styles can help optimize your results. Some popular types of training include:

1. **Strength Training**: This form of training builds muscle mass and is crucial for all body types. It can be beneficial for ectomorphs struggling to gain muscle, endomorphs looking to boost their metabolism, and mesomorphs aiming to maintain their muscle mass. Strength training exercises include free weights, bodyweight exercises, and using resistance machines.
2. **High-Intensity Interval Training (HIIT)**: HIIT is a form of cardiovascular exercise that involves short bursts of high-intensity workouts followed by brief rest

periods. This type of training promotes improvements in endurance and overall fitness while also providing efficient calorie-burning capabilities. HIIT is particularly effective for endomorphs as it helps burn fat and increases metabolism.

3. **Low-Intensity Steady State (LISS)**: LISS is another form of cardiovascular exercise that involves performing activities at a consistent, low-to-moderate intensity for extended periods. This training style is excellent for those starting their fitness journey or for active recovery days. Additionally, LISS can be beneficial for ectomorphs who may struggle with high-intensity exercises, allowing them to burn calories without losing too much muscle mass.

4. **Flexibility and Mobility Training**: Incorporating flexibility and mobility exercises into your workout routine is essential for all body types, improving overall movement and reducing the risk of injury. Focus on stretching and strengthening exercises that target key muscle groups and joints, and consider including activities such as yoga and Pilates.

Adapt Your Nutrition and Recovery Strategies

A tailored fitness routine extends beyond workouts and includes nutrition and recovery strategies that cater to your body's needs. Depending on your goals and body type, you may need to adjust your macronutrient ratios, caloric intake, and meal timing to support muscle gain or fat loss. Prioritize consuming high-quality, nutrient-dense foods to fuel your body for optimal performance and recovery.

Additionally, ensure that you're prioritizing adequate rest and recovery following workouts. This includes incorporating regular rest days, focusing on improving sleep quality, and using recovery techniques such as foam rolling and stress management.

Track Your Progress and Adjust Your Program As Needed

By monitoring your progress, you can objectively evaluate your program's effectiveness and make adjustments based on your body's feedback. Regularly performing assessments, such as body composition measurements, and tracking workout performance metrics will provide you with valuable data to refine your program as needed.

In conclusion, optimizing your fitness routine for your unique body type, goals, and abilities will enable you to achieve optimal health outcomes more efficiently. Consider factors such as body type, training style, nutrition, and rest as crucial components of your tailored workout plan. Don't forget to monitor your progress and adjust your program when needed to keep pushing towards new heights in your fitness journey.

5. Sleep Science: Unveiling the Secrets to Restorative Rest

5.1 The Stages of Sleep and Their Importance

5.1.1 Introduction to Sleep Stages

To understand the science behind sleep, it's essential to learn about the various stages of sleep and their significance in our overall health, cognitive function, and physical performance. Sleep can be categorized into two primary states: **non-rapid eye movement (NREM) sleep** and **rapid eye movement (REM) sleep**. These states, in turn, are divided into a series of stages that recur cyclically throughout our sleep period.

5.1.2 NREM Sleep

NREM sleep is the initial phase of sleep, comprising approximately 75-80% of our total sleep time. This state can be further subdivided into three stages:

- **NREM Stage 1:** This stage is a transitional period between wakefulness and sleep. It's characterized by a shift from beta and gamma brainwave activity— frequencies associated with wakefulness— to slower, more relaxed alpha and theta brainwave patterns. This stage typically lasts for 5-10 minutes, allowing us to drift into a light sleep, where muscles start to relax, and eye movements slow down.
- **NREM Stage 2:** This stage comprises around 45-60% of our total sleep time, and it's during this time that body temperature starts to decrease and heart rate slows down. Brainwave activity continues to transition to slower frequencies– predominantly theta waves– with occasional bursts of rapid, rhythmic brain activity called sleep spindles and sharp, sudden changes in neural activity known as K-complexes.
- **NREM Stage 3:** Commonly referred to as deep, slow-wave sleep (SWS), this stage is marked by the presence of delta brainwave activity, the slowest brainwave frequency that constitutes deep sleep. During this stage, our bodies undergo various

restorative processes essential for muscle growth and repair, immune function, and maintaining hormonal balance. It also plays a crucial role in consolidating and transferring memories from short-term to long-term storage.

5.1.3 REM Sleep

Following the NREM stages, we enter the REM sleep phase, which makes up approximately 20-25% of our sleeping time. The first REM sleep time typically occurs about 90 minutes after falling asleep, and each subsequent REM stage lasts longer than the previous one. REM sleep is marked by several distinct characteristics:

- **Rapid Eye Movements:** As the name suggests, REM sleep is characterized by repeated, rapid, side-to-side eye movements beneath closed eyelids, which can be detected in a sleep study.
- **Vivid Dreaming:** Most of our dreaming occurs during REM sleep, and the dreams tend to be more vivid, bizarre, and emotionally charged.
- **Muscle Atonia:** During this stage, our brain sends inhibitory signals to the spinal cord which temporarily paralyze the muscles in our body, preventing us from physically acting out our dreams, a phenomenon known as REM atonia.
- **Brain Activity and Memory Consolidation:** In REM sleep, brainwave activity resembles the patterns observed during wakefulness, primarily dominated by alpha, beta, and desynchronous brainwaves. This is the stage when our brain consolidates and integrates various forms of information gathered during wakefulness, playing a critical role in learning, problem-solving, and emotion regulation.

5.1.4 Sleep Cycles

Throughout the night, the NREM and REM sleep stages alternate cyclically. A complete sleep cycle typically lasts around 90-120 minutes, comprised of approximately 65-75 minutes of NREM sleep followed by 20-25 minutes of REM sleep.

The distribution of these stages changes as the night progresses. In the early sleep cycles, NREM stage 3 takes up a significant portion of the duration; however, as the night progresses, the duration of Stage 3 sleep declines, with an increase in REM sleep and NREM stage 2 sleep. The longest REM sleep periods usually take place in the later sleep cycles, just before awakening.

5.1.5 The Importance of Sleep Stages

Each sleep stage plays a unique role in optimizing our cognitive and physical health:

- **NREM Stage 1 and 2:** These initial stages help the body and mind transition from wakefulness to sleep and maintain overall sleep continuity throughout the night.
- **NREM Stage 3:** Also known as deep sleep, this stage is critical for physical recovery, cellular regeneration, growth and repair processes, and memory consolidation. Insufficient deep sleep may cause reduced immune function, increased inflammation, impaired glucose metabolism, and reduced cognitive performance.
- **REM Sleep:** This stage is essential for memory consolidation, emotional regulation, and creativity. Insufficient REM sleep may lead to poor learning and memory, emotional disturbances, reduced problem-

solving ability, and an increased risk for mood disorders.

By understanding the intricacies of the sleep stages, we can better appreciate the interconnectedness of these phases in maintaining optimal cognitive function, emotional well-being, and physical health. Consequently, we will be more encouraged to develop and maintain healthy sleep habits and optimally utilize the restorative powers of sleep as an essential element of our biohacking toolkit.

5.1 The Four Sleep Stages: A Journey Through the Night

To completely grasp the concept of restorative sleep, it's crucial first to understand the stages of sleep that our body goes through during a typical night. Sleep can be divided into two main categories: rapid eye movement (REM) sleep and non-REM (NREM) sleep. NREM sleep further consists of three distinct stages: N1, N2, and N3. Our sleep cycles through these stages multiple times a night, roughly every 90 minutes, as we progress from lighter to deeper sleep and finally enter REM sleep.

Let's dive deeper into understanding each sleep stage and its significance.

5.1.1 Stage N1: The Transition Phase

Stage N1, also known as the transition phase, is the lightest stage of sleep. As we drift off from wakefulness, our heart rate, breathing rate, eye movement, and muscle activity begin to slow down. During this stage, we can be easily awakened by sudden sounds or movements. This stage lasts for a brief period, typically 5 to 10 minutes, and accounts for only about 2 to 5% of our total sleep time.

Although brief, the N1 stage is essential for relaxing our body and preparing it for the deeper sleep stages.

5.1.2 Stage N2: Light Sleep

As we enter stage N2, we move from the transition phase to a slightly deeper and more stable state of sleep. Our heart rate and breathing continue to slow down, and our body temperature drops slightly, preparing us for the restorative phase of sleep. During this stage, our muscles continue to relax, and our brain waves exhibit sleep spindles—short bursts of rapid brain activity—indicating that we are truly sleeping.

Stage N2 accounts for approximately 45 to 55% of our total sleep time, and it plays a crucial role in consolidating memories and processing experiences from the day.

5.1.3 Stage N3: Deep Sleep

Stage N3, often referred to as deep sleep or slow-wave sleep, is the most restorative stage of sleep. During this stage, our heart rate, breathing, and brain activity reach their lowest points. Our muscles are completely relaxed, and it becomes difficult to wake us up. This is the stage where the body carries out essential restorative processes, like tissue repair, immune system support, and growth hormone release.

Deep sleep is vital for physical recovery, and it typically accounts for 15 to 25% of our total sleep time. It predominantly occurs during the first half of our sleeping period, and its duration decreases progressively as we age.

5.1.4 REM Sleep: The Dreaming Stage

Approximately 90 minutes after falling asleep, we enter the REM sleep stage. Unlike the previous stages, during REM sleep, our brain activity significantly increases, comparable to the levels of wakefulness. This is the phase where the majority of our dreaming occurs. Our eyes move rapidly from side to side, and our limb muscles become temporarily paralyzed to prevent us from acting out our dreams.

REM sleep is essential for cognitive functions, such as memory consolidation and emotional processing. It accounts for about 20 to 25% of our total sleep time and increases in duration with each subsequent cycle through the night.

5.2 The Importance of Sleep Cycles

Achieving optimal sleep quality and experiencing restorative rest depend on completing multiple sleep cycles and obtaining the right proportions of each sleep stage. Disrupting this cycle can lead to poor sleep quality and reduced overall well-being, even if the total sleep duration remains unchanged.

Biohackers must pay attention to the timing and structure of their sleep cycles in order to maximize the benefits of restorative sleep. Understanding and respecting our body's natural circadian rhythm, or internal sleep-wake cycle, is a key element in optimizing our sleep patterns. This may involve creating a consistent sleep schedule, employing relaxation techniques, and adjusting our sleeping environment to facilitate transition across sleep stages.

By focusing on achieving a balanced and restorative sleep pattern, biohackers can pave the way to improved cognitive functioning, physical performance, and overall well-being in both their waking and sleeping hours.

5.1 Understanding the Sleep Cycle: The Five Stages of Sleep and Their Roles

Before we delve into improving the quality of our sleep, it is essential to understand the sleep cycle and the different stages of sleep. Sleep is a physiological process in which our body and mind can restore and rejuvenate themselves. The sleep cycle, which lasts for about 90 to 110 minutes, comprises five stages: 1, 2, 3, 4, and Rapid Eye Movement (REM) sleep.

Stage 1: Light Sleep (N1)

This is the initial stage when we begin the transition from wakefulness to sleep. At this stage, our brain produces slower brain waves called *alpha* and *theta* waves. Our muscle activity and eye movements also start slowing down. Stage 1 is a relatively brief period, lasting just a few minutes but it is crucial in preparing our body for entering deeper stages of sleep. People awakened during this phase might not even realize they were asleep at all.

Stage 2: Slightly Deeper Sleep (N2)

As we progress into Stage 2, our brain waves continue slowing down with the appearance of *sleep spindles* and *K-complexes*. These two distinct wave patterns are essential for consolidating new memories, learning, and overall cognitive functioning. Our body temperature and heart rate decrease, and our muscle activity further reduces as we enter this stage, which typically constitutes around 45-55% of our sleep.

Stage 3 & 4: Deep Sleep (N3)

Stages 3 and 4 are known as deep sleep or slow-wave sleep (SWS), characterized by the presence of *delta* waves in our brain. Deep sleep is essential for both physical and cognitive restoration. During these stages, our body releases growth hormones that facilitate cell repair, tissue growth, and overall physical recovery. Our immune system also gets replenished at this time. For our mind, deep sleep plays a critical role in memory consolidation, emotion regulation, and cognitive recovery. If you have ever been awakened from deep sleep and felt disoriented, it's because you have been jolted from the restorative magic of these stages.

Stage 5: Rapid Eye Movement (REM) Sleep

REM sleep, typically starting around 90 minutes after we first fall asleep, is the stage where dreams happen. Our body remains paralyzed to prevent us from physically acting out our dreams, while our brain waves speed up, resembling those of an awake state. REM sleep is crucial for processing emotions and memories and plays a significant role in learning and creativity. As the night progresses, the duration of our REM sleep periods increases, with the final one lasting approximately an hour.

Importance of Sleep Cycle Harmony

For optimal health, it is essential to complete multiple sleep cycles throughout the night, cycling through all the stages. Failure to do so results in sleep disruptions and deprivation, which can have significant short-term and long-term consequences.

Short-term consequences of disrupted sleep cycles include:

- Impaired cognitive function and memory

- Mood disturbances, including irritability and anxiety
- Weakened immune system, making you more prone to illness
- Increased risk of accidents and injuries

Long-term consequences of chronic sleep disruptions include:

- Obesity and increased risk of Type 2 diabetes
- Cardiovascular diseases, such as hypertension and heart failure
- Neurological disorders, like Alzheimer's disease and dementia
- Declined mental health, including increased risk of depression and anxiety disorders

In the following sections, we will explore various strategies and biohacks aimed at improving the quality of your sleep by optimizing each stage of the sleep cycle. By making these small yet impactful changes, you can unlock the full potential of restorative rest and significantly improve your overall well-being.

5.1 The Physiology of Sleep: Understanding the Sleep Cycle

Before delving into the methods for optimizing sleep, it is crucial to understand the physiological processes underlying sleep in the human body. This subsection sheds light on the different stages of sleep and the factors that affect sleep quality.

5.1.1 Stages of Sleep

The human brain goes through a series of stages while we sleep, often referred to as the sleep-wake cycle. Sleep researchers have identified four primary stages of sleep, two of which are non-rapid eye movement (NREM) sleep and one of which is rapid eye movement (REM) sleep.

1. **N1 (Stage 1 NREM sleep):** This is a short, transitional phase that occurs when we first drift off to sleep. During this stage, sleep is light, muscles are still active, and we can be easily awakened. Our brain waves slow down, transitioning from wakefulness to sleep. Stage 1 sleep typically lasts for a brief 5 to 10 minutes.
2. **N2 (Stage 2 NREM sleep):** The sleep becomes deeper during this stage, characterized by further relaxation of muscles and a decreased likelihood of being awakened. Brain wave activity continues to slow down, with occasional bursts of quick electrical activity called 'sleep spindles.' N2 sleep typically accounts for 45 to 55% of total sleep time.
3. **N3 (Stage 3 NREM sleep):** Also known as Deep Sleep, Slow-Wave Sleep, or Delta Sleep, this stage is crucial for physical restoration and recovery. During this phase, our brain waves are dominated by slow delta waves, making it difficult to awaken. It is during this stage that the body repairs tissues, builds bone and muscle, and strengthens the immune system. Deep sleep accounts for approximately 20 to 25% of total sleep time.
4. **REM (Rapid Eye Movement) sleep:** This is the stage of sleep where most dreams occur. REM sleep is characterized by rapid eye movements, increased brain activity, and temporary muscle paralysis. This stage is crucial for learning, memory consolidation, and cognitive function. During REM sleep, the brain processes and stores new information, making

connections with previously stored knowledge. REM sleep accounts for approximately 20 to 25% of total sleep time.

The sleep cycle progresses cyclically through these different sleep stages multiple times throughout the night, with each cycle lasting approximately 90 minutes. Each subsequent cycle contains less deep sleep (N3) and more REM sleep.

5.1.2 The Circadian Rhythm and Sleep Regulation

Sleep is regulated by two primary mechanisms: the circadian rhythm and sleep-wake homeostasis.

- **Circadian rhythm:** Often referred to as the 'body clock,' the circadian rhythm is a natural, internal cycle that regulates the timing of sleep and wakefulness. The hypothalamus, a small region in the brain, controls the circadian rhythm by responding to environmental cues such as light and darkness. Exposure to natural light during the day supports a healthy circadian rhythm and promotes better sleep at night.
- **Sleep-wake homeostasis:** This is the body's internal sleep drive, which balances sleep and wakefulness by maintaining a 'sleep debt' that gets accumulated during wakefulness. As we stay awake for longer, our urge to sleep increases. Ideally, this sleep debt should be 'paid off' by sufficient sleep each night.

5.1.3 Factors Affecting Sleep Quality

Several factors can interfere with the natural sleep cycle, affecting the sleep quality:

- **Light exposure:** Exposure to artificial light, particularly blue light from screens, can disrupt the circadian rhythm and suppress the production of the sleep hormone melatonin, leading to difficulty falling asleep and reduced sleep quality.
- **Stress and anxiety:** High stress levels and anxiety can make it difficult to relax and fall asleep. Additionally, the racing thoughts associated with anxiety can also cause nighttime awakenings and disrupt sleep.
- **Diet:** The consumption of stimulating food and drink, such as caffeine and sugar, particularly in the few hours leading up to bedtime, can interfere with our ability to fall asleep and stay asleep.
- **Exercise:** Engaging in regular physical activity is known to promote better sleep; however, doing strenuous exercise too close to bedtime can potentially interfere with the natural sleep cycle.
- **Sleep environment:** A sleep environment that is too hot, too cold, noisy or uncomfortable can adversely affect sleep quality. Creating a comfortable, dark, and quiet sleep space is vital for promoting restorative sleep.

In the following subsections, we will explore various biohacking strategies to optimize each aspect of the sleep cycle and create an ideal environment for restorative sleep. From improving sleep hygiene to enhancing our sleep environment, we will unveil the most effective ways to hack your sleep and unlock the full potential of this vital aspect of health and well-being.

5.1 Understand the Sleep Cycles: A Guide to Decoding the Biological Rhythms

A good night's sleep is crucial for maintaining optimal health, but despite spending roughly one-third of our lives sleeping, most of us don't fully understand the intricacies of our biological sleep patterns. In this section, we will explore the different stages of sleep, how our bodies cycle through these phases, and the processes that occur during each one. Understanding these cycles is essential for biohackers looking to optimize their sleep and overall wellbeing.

The Science of Sleep: *Circadian Rhythm*

At the root of our sleep patterns is the circadian rhythm, a biological process that regulates our body's internal clock. This clock influences a multitude of bodily functions, including sleep-wake cycles, hormone release, body temperature, and digestion. Disruptions to the circadian rhythm, commonly known as jet lag or shift work sleep disorder, can lead to sleep disturbances, mood changes, and weakened immune systems.

It is important for biohackers to maintain a consistent sleep schedule that aligns with their circadian rhythm. Doing so will help promote restorative sleep and encourage optimal cognitive and physical functioning.

The Stages of Sleep: *NREM and REM Cycles*

Sleep is divided into two broad categories: *non-rapid eye movement (NREM)* sleep and *rapid eye movement (REM)* sleep. These two categories are further broken down into a series of distinct stages that make up the sleep cycle. During a typical night, we cycle through these stages approximately 4-6 times, with each cycle lasting about 90 minutes.

Stage 1: Light Sleep (NREM)

Stage 1 is the initial phase of sleep, also called light sleep. This stage typically lasts for a few minutes and serves as a transition from wakefulness to deeper sleep. Muscle activity begins to slow, the heart rate and breathing become regulated, and the body begins to relax. This is the stage where you may experience sudden muscle twitches or a sensation of falling, known as hypnic jerks.

Stage 2: Intermediate Sleep (NREM)

Following stage 1, we transition into stage 2, which is still considered light sleep, but with some physiological changes taking place. Brainwaves slow down, body temperature decreases, and heart rate and blood pressure reduce further. It is during this stage that the body begins to repair itself and strengthen the immune system. Stage 2 typically makes up the majority of our sleep each night.

Stage 3: Deep Sleep (NREM)

Stage 3 is deep, restorative sleep. During this stage, the body undergoes significant restoration and growth processes. Muscles relax, blood vessels dilate, and blood flow to muscles increases. Human growth hormone is released, which promotes cell growth and repair, and the immune system works to combat infections and inflammation. Additionally, Stage 3 sleep plays a crucial role in consolidating and processing information from the day, building long-term memories, and enhancing cognitive functioning.

The final stage of the sleep cycle is characterized by rapid eye movement, increased brain activity, and vivid dreams. REM sleep is essential for cognitive functions such as learning, memory consolidation, and emotional processing. During this stage, the body is relatively still due to temporary muscle paralysis, which is thought to prevent us from physically acting out our dreams.

Biohacking Tips for Better Sleep:

Understanding the science of sleep and how it impacts our overall health is essential for biohackers looking to optimize their wellbeing. Here are some biohacking tips designed to promote restorative sleep and improve overall health:

1. **Maintain a consistent sleep schedule:** Going to bed and waking up at the same time each day helps to regulate your circadian rhythm, ensuring a better quality of sleep and enhanced daytime functioning.
2. **Create an optimal sleep environment:** Make your bedroom a sleep sanctuary by blocking out excess light, maintaining a cool temperature, and limiting noise disturbances.
3. **Optimize your evening routine:** Establish a relaxing bedtime routine that includes activities such as reading, gentle stretching, or meditation to signal to your body that it is time for sleep.
4. **Monitor sleep quality and quantity:** Use a sleep tracking device or app to better understand your sleep patterns and make adjustments as needed.
5. **Be mindful of your diet and exercise:** Eating a balanced diet, avoiding stimulants like caffeine before bed, and engaging in regular physical activity can all contribute to a better night's sleep.

By gaining a deeper understanding of the science behind our sleep cycles and taking proactive steps to optimize our sleep environment and routines, we can unlock the true potential of restorative rest and improve overall health and wellbeing.

6. Stress Management: The Art of Resilience and Tapping into Flow States

The Art of Resilience: How to Bounce Back Stronger Than Before

Resilience is the ability to adapt positively in the face of stress, adversity, and change. It is the capacity to recover quickly from difficulties and maintain our emotional, mental, and physical well-being. In a world where stress is inevitable, developing resilience becomes crucial to ensure not only survival but also leading a healthy, productive, and fulfilling life.

The Components of Resilience: Building a Foundation

Research has identified several key components that contribute to building resilience. Understanding and integrating these components will help you develop the skills and mindset necessary to bounce back stronger than before.

1. **Emotional intelligence**: Emotional intelligence refers to the ability to recognize, understand, and manage our own emotions as well as empathize with and

respond constructively to the emotions of others. Emotionally intelligent individuals can adapt better to stressful situations and communicate effectively with others, which are integral elements of resilience.

2. **Situational awareness**: This means being able to accurately assess your environment and identify potential stressors before they become overwhelming. By staying aware of your surroundings and making necessary adjustments to your mindset or approach, you can minimize the impact of stress on your well-being.

3. **Personal responsibility**: Taking personal responsibility for your actions, thoughts, and emotions is an essential aspect of resilience. By acknowledging that you have control over your reactions and choices, you can develop the ability to take charge of your life, no matter the circumstances.

4. **Realistic optimism**: While it is essential to maintain a positive outlook on life, being overly optimistic can be detrimental. Adopting a balanced perspective that acknowledges both the positive and negative aspects of a situation will help you maintain a healthy level of optimism and resilience.

5. **Strong support network**: Building and maintaining a robust network of support, comprised of friends, family, and colleagues, is essential for resilience. When faced with adversity, you can lean on your support system for encouragement, guidance, and understanding, helping you develop the strength needed to bounce back.

Tapping into Flow States for Enhanced Stress Management

A "flow state" is the mental state in which an individual is fully immersed in an activity, experiencing a sense of energized focus, full involvement, and enjoyment. Achieving a flow state can lead to an increased sense of well-being and performance, reducing the impact of stress on our lives.

To tap into flow states and optimize your stress management, follow these steps:

1. **Find your passion**: Flow generally occurs when you engage in activities that you genuinely enjoy and find meaningful. Identify your passions, hobbies, or areas of interest in your life, and make time to indulge in these activities regularly.
2. **Set clear, achievable goals**: Clarity in your objectives is essential for entering the flow state. Ensure that your goals are well-defined and attainable within the context of the activity.
3. **Seek challenges and embrace growth**: Flow states can be reached when you challenge your abilities, pushing yourself outside your comfort zone while remaining within your skill level. Strive for gradual, achievable growth in your chosen activity.
4. **Cultivate focus and mindfulness**: Enhance your ability to concentrate and be present during an activity by practicing mindfulness techniques such as meditation, deep breathing, or progressive muscle relaxation.
5. **Minimize distractions**: Create an environment that minimizes distractions and allows you to focus fully on the task at hand. This could include creating a designated workspace, implementing a routine, or utilizing noise-canceling headphones.
6. **Monitor your progress**: Assess your progress and performance during the activity, adjusting your approach or techniques if necessary. Maintain a healthy relationship with feedback, seeing setbacks as opportunities for learning and growth.

7. **Practice patience and persistence**: Achieving a flow state takes time, so be patient with yourself and persistently engage in activities you enjoy. As you practice, you will become more adept at tapping into flow states, enhancing your ability to manage stress.

By developing resilience and learning to tap into flow states, you can effectively manage stress, optimize your well-being, and lead a more fulfilling life. Remember, stress is an inevitable part of life, but how we respond to it is entirely within our control. Embrace the challenge, and take a proactive approach to stress management by honing your resilience and welcoming flow in your daily life.

6.1 Understanding Stress and Its Impact on Health

Before diving into stress management techniques and strategies to achieve flow states, it's essential to understand what stress is and how it affects our health. Simply put, stress is the body's response to perceived threats or challenges. The human brain releases stress hormones such as cortisol and adrenaline in reaction to stress, preparing the body to either fight or flee the perceived danger.

While stress is a natural and necessary part of life, chronic stress can lead to or exacerbate several health issues, including mental health problems such as anxiety and depression, poor immune function, and chronic illnesses like heart disease and diabetes. Understanding how stress impacts our well-being is crucial in our pursuit of optimal health.

The Types of Stress

Stress can be divided into three main categories- acute, chronic, and eustress. Each type of stress affects the body differently and requires different management approaches for promoting resilience and tapping into flow states.

- **Acute stress**: This short-term stress is caused by immediate threats, challenges, or demands. It's often intense but brief, producing an immediate physiological response. Once the threat has passed or is resolved, the body usually returns to its normal state. Examples of acute stress could be a job interview, a sports event, or even an intense workout. While acute stress can be unpleasant, it can also be helpful in pushing individuals to perform under pressure.
- **Chronic stress**: Unlike acute stress, chronic stress is long-term and persistent, negatively affecting overall health and well-being. Prolonged exposure to stress can result in high cortisol levels and a weakened immune system, increasing the risk of mental and physical health issues. Examples of chronic stress could be ongoing financial strain, relationship troubles, or dissatisfaction with one's work-life balance.
- **Eustress**: This type of stress is typically seen as positive or helpful. Eustress pushes individuals to grow and develop, motivating them towards an improved sense of well-being. Examples of eustress include working on a passion project, getting married, or challenging oneself with a new skill or hobby.

Building Resilience and Managing Stress

Resilience refers to the ability to adapt and recover after experiencing stressful situations. Cultivating resilience can help you manage stress and prevent it from negatively impacting your health. By incorporating resilience-building practices into your life, you can reduce the effects of both acute and chronic stress and unlock greater overall well-being.

1. **Mindfulness Meditation:** Practicing mindfulness meditation can help you become more aware of your thoughts, emotions, and sensations in the present moment. This heightened awareness can help you better manage stress by allowing you to identify it, understand its causes, and respond to it in a healthier way.
2. **Social Support:** Strengthening relationships and building connections can provide much-needed support during stressful times. Reach out to friends, family, or support groups in times of need and nurture relationships that bring positivity and laughter into your life.
3. **Exercise:** Regular physical activity not only improves overall health but also promotes mental wellness by releasing endorphins, which are natural stress reducers. Exercise can also serve as a means of stress relief, taking your mind off your concerns and helping you feel more connected to your body.
4. **Sleep:** Good sleep hygiene is crucial for managing stress and building resilience. Ensure that you're getting adequate rest and maintaining a consistent sleep schedule to allow your body and mind to properly recover.
5. **Emotional Intelligence:** Improving emotional intelligence can help you better understand, manage, and regulate your emotions. Understanding your emotions is a vital component of stress management, as it allows you to respond to stressors in a healthier, more adaptive way.

Tapping into Flow States for Optimal Performance

A flow state, also referred to as "being in the zone," is a psychological state in which individuals are fully absorbed in a challenging activity, losing themselves in the task at hand. Flow states lead to optimal performance and a sense of enjoyment of the task, offering a powerful antidote to stress.

Achieving a flow state involves finding the sweet spot between challenge and skill, where the demands of the task match your abilities. To tap into flow states and maintain them, consider the following strategies:

1. **Set Clear Goals**: Having clear, achievable goals can help create a sense of purpose and motivate you towards your objectives.
2. **Develop Your Skills**: Continually hone your skills to match the demands of your tasks. This might involve learning from mentors, seeking feedback, or engaging in deliberate practice.
3. **Eliminate Distractions**: Remove any distractions that might impede your ability to focus on the task at hand. This might involve setting up a clutter-free work environment, turning off notifications on electronic devices, or establishing designated work times.
4. **Cultivate Positive Mindsets**: Be open to new experiences, maintain a curiosity for learning, and foster a growth mindset to build your resilience and ability to achieve flow states.

In summary, managing stress, building resilience, and tapping into flow states can play a crucial role in achieving optimal health. By understanding the different types of stress, incorporating resilience-building practices, and cultivating strategies to access flow states, you can harness the power of your body and mind to achieve your full potential.

6.1 Understanding Stress and Its Impact on Optimal Health

Stress is an inevitable part of our modern lives, and our understanding of it has evolved significantly over the past century. Once construed as a purely negative force, stress is now believed to have room for positive adaptation depending on the circumstances, duration, and intensity. In this section, we will explore the nature of stress, how it impacts our health, and the importance of developing resilience and tapping into flow states to achieve biohacker's optimal health.

Acute versus Chronic Stress

Stress primarily falls into two categories - acute and chronic. Acute stress results from short-lived, immediate events that trigger our 'fight or flight' response. Events like narrowly avoiding a car accident or taking a challenging test are examples of acute stressors. These acute stressors can actually benefit us by heightening our focus and preparing us for action.

On the other hand, chronic stress results from long-term challenges or situations that require continuous effort and attention. Chronic stress can stem from work-related issues, financial difficulties, a tumultuous relationship, or even a persistently negative mindset. It is this chronic stress that poses the greatest threat to our optimal health, as it can lead to physical, mental, and emotional imbalances.

Consequences of Unmanaged Chronic Stress

If chronic stress is not managed or relieved, it can result in harmful consequences, including:

1. **Hormonal Imbalances**: Chronic stress can throw our body's hormonal balance off-kilter, causing a potentially destructive cycle of hormonal imbalances, including elevated cortisol levels, which can lead to visceral fat accumulation, impaired cognitive function, and increased risk for chronic diseases.
2. **Immunosuppression**: Chronic stress weakens our immune system, thereby increasing susceptibility to infections and illness over time.
3. **Mental Health Disorders**: Prolonged exposure to chronic stress can contribute to mental health issues, such as anxiety and depression.
4. **Sleep Disturbances**: Our ability to enjoy restful, restorative sleep can be severely hampered by persistent stress.
5. **Chronic Inflammation**: Chronic stress may lead to long-lasting inflammation within the body, which is associated with various chronic ailments, including heart disease and diabetes.

6.1.1 Building Resilience: Strategies for Battling Stress

While it's impossible to eliminate all stress from our lives, enhancing your resilience to stress is within your control. Building resilience is a key component of biohackers' pursuit of optimal health, as it enables us to cope more effectively with everyday stressors and the more significant challenges that life may throw at us.

Here are some strategies to help you build resilience:

1. **Cultivate a Positive Mindset**: Focus on developing an optimistic outlook on life and embrace a growth mindset, which encourages learning from failures and setbacks.

2. **Establish a Support Network**: Nurture social connections with friends and family, as well as seek out communities and support groups where you can share your experiences and cultivate connections.
3. **Engage in Regular Exercise**: Physical activity helps regulate stress hormones and release feel-good endorphins, which promote mental well-being.
4. **Practice Mindfulness**: Adopting mindfulness practices, such as meditation and yoga, can help you manage stress, become more present, and develop compassion for yourself and others.
5. **Prioritize Proper Sleep Hygiene**: Ensure you are meeting your body's sleep needs by establishing a consistent sleep routine and optimizing your sleep environment.
6. **Develop Coping Mechanisms**: Develop healthy coping mechanisms to deal with stress, such as humor, journaling, or seeking professional help when needed.

6.1.2 Tapping into Flow States

Flow states, coined by psychologist Mihaly Csikszentmihalyi, describe a peak state where individuals experience complete absorption in the task at hand, a heightened sense of focus, and optimal productivity. Flow states can contribute to stress management by removing external distractions, promoting creativity and innovation, and increasing overall well-being.

To tap into flow states, consider the following elements necessary to induce flow:

1. **Clear Goals**: Set clear, attainable goals for the task at hand, so you know exactly what is expected.

2. **Immediate Feedback**: Timely feedback helps you adjust your performance accordingly and maintain momentum.
3. **Challenging but Achievable**: Engage in activities that require a balance between your skills and the challenge presented. Tasks that are too simple result in boredom, while overly complex tasks may lead to anxiety.
4. **Focused Concentration**: Minimize distractions and give yourself permission to immerse yourself fully in the task.
5. **Control**: Establish a sense of control over the activity by gaining the necessary skills and knowledge.
6. **Enjoyment**: Choose activities that are intrinsically rewarding and enjoyable for you.

By developing resilience and tapping into flow states, you can effectively harness stress as a beneficial force, rather than allowing it to undermine your pursuit of optimal health. Practicing these techniques can set the stage for improved wellness and vitality, making them essential components of a successful biohacking journey.

6.1 The Synergy of Stress and Resilience: The Path to Optimal Performance

It is essential to understand the intricate relationship between stress and resilience to grasp how to manage and cope with the challenges that life presents. The more resilient one becomes, the higher their resistance to stress, making it imperative to foster both simultaneously. This synergy is not just about preventing chronic stress or burnout; it is also about enhancing well-being, unlocking fluidity in day-to-day experiences, and increasing overall cognitive and physical performance.

Understanding Stress and Resilience

Stress can be defined as a physical, mental, or emotional strain or tension resulting from demanding circumstances. Stress is an integral part of life and can be categorized into two categories: acute stress and chronic stress. Acute stress is short-term and can be beneficial in certain situations, such as increased alertness and focus during a presentation or athletic event. Chronic stress, on the other hand, is long-term and has detrimental impacts on mental and physical health.

Resilience is the ability to adapt and bounce back from adversity, trauma, or stress. It is a dynamic process involving a complex interaction between individual and environmental factors. Developing one's resilience can provide numerous benefits such as improved mental health, increased productivity, and better overall quality of life.

Components of Resilience

Resilience is multifaceted and can be cultivated on different levels: personal, emotional, cognitive, and physical. Some key components of resilience include:

1. **Personal resilience**: Involves aspects such as self-awareness, personal values, and a growth mindset. Cultivating personal resilience means building better self-esteem, self-compassion, and a more robust sense of purpose.
2. **Emotional resilience**: Encompasses the ability to regulate and adapt one's emotions during difficult situations. Building emotional resilience entails

increasing emotional intelligence, practicing mindfulness, and developing healthy coping mechanisms.

3. **Cognitive resilience**: Entails the capacity to rationally process and manage stressors, make effective decisions, and solve problems. Building cognitive resilience involves strengthening skills such as critical thinking, cognitive flexibility, and mental stamina.

4. **Physical resilience**: Relates to the body's ability to withstand and recover from physical stressors. Physical resilience can be built through regular exercise, proper nutrition, and sufficient sleep.

Practices to Build Resilience and Manage Stress

There are several practical strategies one can adapt or use to improve resilience and stress management:

1. Develop a Growth Mindset: Embrace the idea that challenges and failures are part of the learning and growing process. With a growth mindset, one can perceive adversity as an opportunity for self-improvement rather than a setback.

2. Cultivate Self-Compassion: To build resilience, practice being kind and understanding toward oneself when facing setbacks. Replace negative self-talk with positive, realistic self-affirmations.

3. Foster a Support Network: Having a strong support network can enhance feelings of safety, improve problem-solving strategies, and contribute to overall resilience. Engage regularly in social interactions and maintain healthy relationships with friends, family, and mentors.

4. Mindfulness Meditation: By practicing mindfulness, one can reduce stress by staying present and accepting one's thoughts and emotions. This practice helps individuals manage their reactions to stress and improve emotional resilience.

5. Commit to Regular Physical Activity: Engage in regular physical exercise to enhance overall well-being, reduce stress levels, and increase energy. Physical activity not only helps to build physical resilience but also supports cognitive and emotional well-being.

6. Prioritize Self-Care: Establish a self-care routine that focuses on mental, physical, and emotional well-being. This routine may consist of activities such as enjoying hobbies, spending quality time with loved ones, or taking time to relax and recharge.

7. Develop Healthy Sleeping Habits: Prioritize obtaining adequate, quality sleep to bolster physical and mental resilience. Establish a consistent sleep schedule and create an environment conducive to restful slumber.

Tapping into Flow States

A flow state, also known as being "in the zone," is a mental state in which an individual is fully immersed in an activity, experiencing a sense of heightened focus, energy, and enjoyment. Flow states have been associated with higher performance, improved creativity, and enhanced well-being.

To tap into flow states, consider adopting the following practices:

1. **Identify Passion-Driven Activities**: Engage in tasks that spark excitement, curiosity, or genuine interest, which increase the likelihood of experiencing flow.

2. **Set Clear Goals**: Define explicit objectives that are challenging but achievable. Ensure one's goals provide structure and direction during an activity.
3. **Eliminate Distractions**: Create an environment free from interruptions and distractions to facilitate concentration and focused attention.
4. **Establish a Balance between Skill Level and Challenge**: Maintain sufficient challenges without overpowering one's skillset. This balance adds a sense of control and mastery, enhancing the flow experience.
5. **Prioritize Immediate Feedback**: Engage in activities where instantaneous feedback is available, ensuring that one can align efforts and outcomes, adjust behaviors, and track progress.

The synergy between stress, resilience, and flow states play a crucial role in contributing to one's overall health and well-being. By implementing practices to enhance resilience, manage stress, and tap into flow states, individuals can unlock their potential for improved mental, emotional, and physical performance.

6.1 The Role of Stress in Our Lives and the Importance of Resilience

In today's fast-paced, high-pressure world, stress is an inevitable part of our daily lives. Many of us juggle multiple roles and responsibilities - such as work, interpersonal relationships, and health goals - leaving us susceptible to stressors that can negatively impact our well-being. The way we cope with stress can have a significant influence on our overall physical, mental, and emotional health. But why exactly is stress so detrimental, and how can we foster resilience to better manage it?

Stress: The Good, The Bad, and the Ugly

Believe it or not, stress is not entirely bad. A certain level of stress is actually beneficial to us. When experiencing a challenging situation, our bodies release stress hormones such as cortisol and adrenaline that prepare us to either face the challenge head-on or retreat to safety. This natural biological response, known as the "fight or flight" response, serves the purpose of enhancing our survival as a species.

However, the issue arises when we face chronic stress. Prolonged exposure to stress without adequate time for recovery can lead to various negative physiological and psychological outcomes. Chronically high cortisol levels have been associated with numerous health issues, such as weakened immune function, weight gain, and heart disease. Furthermore, we are more susceptible to mental health issues like anxiety, depression, and burnout when we are constantly under stress.

Building Resilience: Key Strategies for Stress Management

Resilience refers to our ability to adapt and recover from adversity and stress. It is a crucial skill to develop if we wish to maintain peak physical, mental, and emotional well-being in the face of our hectic modern lifestyles. Here are several strategies that can help you build resilience and better manage stress:

1. **Mindfulness and Meditation:** One major component of resilience is our ability to remain aware and present in the face of challenges. Mindfulness and meditation practices help us cultivate this awareness and subsequently facilitate more effective stress management. By consciously acknowledging our

stressors and current emotional state, we can develop healthier strategies for coping with stress rather than resorting to unhealthy patterns of behavior.

2. **Physical Activity:** Engaging in regular physical activity is essential for stress reduction and resilience-building. Exercise has been shown to have a multitude of benefits to mental health, including decreased stress levels, improved mood, and increased production of neurochemicals like endorphins and serotonin. Choose an activity you enjoy, such as running, lifting weights, or yoga, and aim to incorporate it into your regular routine.

3. **Social Support:** Our connections with others play a major role in our ability to weather life's challenges. Strong social networks provide a sense of belonging, which can increase feelings of self-worth and emotional resilience. Make an effort to maintain and nurture your relationships with friends, family, and other support systems to foster deeper connections and enhanced resilience.

4. **Optimal Sleep:** Prioritizing quality sleep is another integral aspect of stress management. When we don't get adequate rest, our bodies' ability to cope with stress dips significantly, leaving us more vulnerable to the negative effects of chronic stress. Focus on building healthy sleep habits, such as maintaining a consistent sleep schedule, creating a relaxing bedtime routine, and ensuring your sleep environment is conducive to restful slumber.

5. **Cognitive Flexibility:** Having the ability to adapt our thoughts and change our perspectives when faced with new circumstances is crucial for resilience. Developing cognitive flexibility can help us handle stressors more effectively and prevent rumination or negative thought patterns that compound stress. Techniques such as cognitive behavioral therapy and

practicing self-compassion can help us adjust our thought patterns and promote cognitive flexibility.

6.2 Tapping into Flow States: Unleashing Our Inner Potential

The concept of "flow states," coined by psychologist Mihaly Csikszentmihalyi, refers to a state of optimal experience and heightened focus during which we are fully absorbed in the task at hand. During a flow state, our sense of time may become distorted, our awareness of ourselves dissipates, and our performance is elevated to new heights. This potent state has been linked to increased creativity, problem-solving abilities, and overall well-being. By learning to tap into flow states, we can not only achieve better stress management, but also unleash our inner potential.

Entering the Flow State: Key Elements

To access flow states, it is essential to create the right conditions for them to occur. Here are several key elements required for entering into flow:

1. **Challenge-Skills Balance:** Flow occurs when we are engaged in an activity that presents an appropriate level of challenge, one that is neither too easy nor too difficult. If the task is too simple, we may become bored and disengage; if it's too difficult, we may become overwhelmed and anxious, thwarting the possibility of flow. Seek activities that strike the perfect balance to optimize your chances of experiencing flow.
2. **Clear Goals and Immediate Feedback:** Having a clear objective and receiving immediate feedback on

progress allow us to focus on the process and fine-tune our engagement with the task. This in turn supports the development of the flow state.

3. **Concentration and Focus:** Flow states require deep mental engagement and a laser-like focus on the task at hand. Eliminate any distractions to help maintain this level of concentration. This may involve creating a conducive environment, using techniques like deep work or the Pomodoro technique, and ensuring your mind is well-rested.

4. **Intrinsic Motivation and Enjoyment:** Engaging in tasks we are intrinsically motivated to perform and genuinely enjoy can increase our likelihood of entering flow states. Foster your passion for activities that challenge and stimulate you, as these are more likely to induce flow.

By incorporating these elements and actively seeking out activities that facilitate flow, we can unlock the door to heightened focus, creativity, and overall well-being in our lives. Not only will we find our capacity to manage stress significantly elevated, but we will also experience a newfound sense of fulfillment and personal growth. Through cultivating resilience and embracing flow states, we build a foundation of optimal health that empowers us to live our lives to the fullest.

7. Environmental Adaptation: Shaping Your Space for Health and Longevity

7.1 The Art of Designing Your Space: Principles for Health and Longevity

While the concept of biohacking largely revolves around making adjustments to your natural physiology and genetics, designing an environment that supports and enhances your health is equally important. In this rapidly changing world, our spaces have the power to impact our health in numerous ways, from the air we breathe to the amount of natural light we receive. In this chapter, we will explore several principles for shaping the spaces you inhabit in a way that promotes health and longevity.

7.1.1 Biophilic Design: Embracing Our Connection to Nature

Human beings have evolved in and around natural environments over thousands of years, and our innate bond with the natural world is something many of us cannot ignore. Biophilic design is an approach to architectural and interior design that incorporates natural elements into modern spaces to improve the health and wellbeing of inhabitants. Some ways to incorporate biophilic design into your environment include:

1. **Natural Light**: Make the most of natural lighting by ensuring your space has ample windows and skylights. Arrange your furniture in such a way that you receive the most sunlight throughout the day. Regular exposure to daylight helps regulate your circadian rhythm and can help improve mood and sleep quality.

2. **Green Spaces**: Add indoor plants to your space, or design a green wall or vertical garden. Plants not only improve air quality by absorbing pollutants and releasing oxygen but can also have positive psychological effects, reducing stress and aiding concentration.
3. **Natural Materials**: Use furnishings and finishes made of natural materials like wood, stone, and bamboo. Natural textures and patterns can have a calming effect and create a sense of connection to the outdoors.
4. **Biodynamic Lighting**: Install dynamic lighting systems that mimic the fluctuations of sunlight throughout the day. This can help regulate your circadian rhythm and support optimal energy levels.
5. **Nature-Inspired Art**: Decorate your space with art or patterns inspired by nature. Research has shown that even simulated representations of nature can have a positive impact on mood and stress levels.

7.1.2 Ergonomic Spaces: Respecting the Human Body's Design

Ergonomics is the science of adapting your environment to the way your body moves and functions, in order to reduce discomfort, strain, and potential injury. This principle can be applied to the spaces we live and work in, with the following considerations:

1. **Workspace Ergonomics**: Ensure your office and work setup supports healthy posture and reduces the strain on your spine, neck, and shoulders. Invest in an adjustable-chair, ensure your computer monitor is at the correct height, and consider using ergonomic accessories such as a split keyboard and a vertical mouse.

2. **Movement-Oriented Spaces**: Design your space in such a way that encourages movement and walking. For example, create a layout with multiple activity zones, place items you frequently use in different areas, or set up a standing desk to provide an alternative to sitting for long durations.
3. **Restorative Spaces**: Create spaces in your environment that encourage rest and relaxation. This could include a cozy reading nook, a meditation area, or a designated space for stretching or practicing yoga.

7.1.3 Air Quality and Health: Breathing Easier Indoors

Indoor air quality can have a significant impact on our health, particularly as we spend a majority of our time indoors. To improve the air quality in your environment:

1. **Ventilation**: Ensure that your space has sufficient ventilation by regularly opening windows, installing an air exchange system, or using air purifiers with HEPA filters to remove contaminants and allergens.
2. **Eliminate VOCs**: Volatile organic compounds (VOCs) are emitted as gases from certain solids or liquids, such as paints, building materials, and cleaning products. Opt for low or zero-VOC products to minimize their presence in your environment.
3. **Humidity Control**: Maintain a healthy level of indoor humidity, often between 30-50%. This can help prevent the growth of mold and dust mites, which can cause allergies and respiratory issues. Invest in a humidifier or dehumidifier if needed.

7.1.4 Acoustic Comfort: Reducing Noise and Enhancing Wellness

Noise pollution can have a significant impact on our health, contributing to stress, sleep disruption, and even cardiovascular issues. To create a more acoustically comfortable space:

1. **Sound Proofing**: Utilize materials and building techniques that help reduce the transmission of sound between spaces, such as insulation, acoustic panels, or double-glazing windows.
2. **Noise-Reducing Materials**: Opt for soft furnishings and materials that absorb sound, such as curtains, upholstered furniture, and rugs. These can help reduce echo and unwanted noise in your environment.
3. **Nature Sounds**: Introduce calming sounds of nature, such as a water feature or a white noise machine, to create an ambiance that promotes relaxation and stress reduction.

By considering these principles when designing your space, you can effectively turn your environment into an ally in your pursuit of optimal health and longevity, supporting and enhancing the effects of your other biohacking efforts.

7.2 Environmental Ergonomics: Designing Spaces for Movement and Posture

A vital aspect of environmental adaptation is the intentional design of spaces that encourage **movement and proper body posture**. By optimizing our surroundings for better health and longevity, we create an environment that reinforces positive habits and discourages sedentary behavior. This section focuses on strategies to shape your workspace, home, and everyday environment for optimal health.

7.2.1 Transforming the Workspace

The rise of sedentary lifestyles and the increase in remote work have highlighted the importance of having an environment that promotes movement and good posture. Here are some ways to modify your workspace to encourage healthy habits:

- **Adjustable Desks**: Consider investing in a height-adjustable standing desk or a desk converter that allows you to alternate between sitting and standing throughout the day. Standing desks can help reduce the risks associated with prolonged sitting, such as obesity, heart disease, and diabetes.
- **Ergonomic Chairs**: Select a chair that provides proper lumbar support, encourages good posture, and can be adjusted to a comfortable height. Ergonomic chairs can alleviate the strain on the lower back, reduce the risk of developing musculoskeletal disorders, and improve overall well-being.
- **Monitor Placement**: Position your computer monitor at eye level and about 20-30 inches away from your eyes. This can reduce eye strain, headaches, and neck tension, and also promote proper head posture.
- **Keyboard and Mouse**: Choose ergonomic keyboard and mouse designs that minimize strain on the wrists and hands. For added comfort, use a padded wrist rest.
- **Movement Breaks**: Integrate movement activities into your daily schedule. Set a timer to remind you to

take regular breaks throughout the day to stand, walk, stretch, or perform other physical activities.

7.2.2 Designing a Movement-friendly Home

Your home environment can also be optimized for better health and longevity. Here we present a few ideas on how to create a space that encourages movement and mindful living:

- **Activity Zones**: Designate specific areas within your home for various activities, such as yoga, meditation, or exercise. Having dedicated zones can help create a natural flow of movement and remind you to engage in regular physical activities.
- **Workout Equipment**: Make fitness equipment easily accessible in your daily environment. For example, keep a set of resistance bands within reach, or set up a pull-up bar in a doorway. Having the equipment readily available can increase the likelihood of engaging in spontaneous workouts.
- **Furniture Arrangement**: Arrange your furniture in a way that encourages movement and interaction. For example, setting your sofa a slight distance from a coffee table might encourage you to stand up and stretch whenever you reach for an item.
- **Stair Use**: If you have stairs in your home or building, commit to using them instead of taking the elevator, as it is an easy way to incorporate more physical activity into your day.
- **Decluttered Spaces**: Keep your living space free from clutter to prevent tripping hazards and promote a peaceful, mindful environment. By maintaining a clean space, you create a comfortable environment for movement and relaxation.

7.2.3 Daily Environment Adaptation

Environmental adaptation is a continuous process, and minor alterations in our daily environments can lead to significant improvements in our health and longevity. Some practical ideas include:

- **Walking or Biking**: Implement walking or biking as part of your daily routine, whether it be for commuting to work, doing errands, or engaging in recreational activities.
- **Public Spaces**: Make use of public recreational areas, such as parks, walking trails, or community centers, to enjoy outdoor activities and connect with nature.
- **Social Interaction**: Encourage in-person social interactions by participating in group activities, exercise classes, or joining local interest clubs. Social connections can motivate us to stay active and engaged in our environment.
- **Adopt a Pet**: Adopting a pet, like a dog, can encourage regular walks and outdoor play, providing not only physical benefits but also emotional ones.

In conclusion, by intentionally considering the design of our working, living, and daily environments, we can foster healthier habits, promote better posture, and enhance overall wellness. The power of environmental adaptation lies in its capacity to shape our behavior and create spaces that support our pursuit of optimal health and longevity. By proactively adapting our environment, we set the foundation for a healthier and more active lifestyle.

7. Environmental Adaptation: Shaping Your Space for Health and Longevity

Our environment plays a significant role in our overall health and well-being. It is essential that we recognize and harness the power of our surroundings to optimize our physical and mental health. In this section, we will delve into various strategies for adapting and shaping our environment to promote overall health and longevity.

7.1 The Healing Impact of Natural Light

Exposure to natural light is greatly beneficial for our health. Not only does it set our circadian rhythm, our body's internal clock, but it also supports our mental wellbeing, productivity, and sleep quality. Here are some ways to increase your exposure to natural light:

- Open your curtains or blinds during daytime hours to let in as much sunlight as possible.
- Move your workspace or sitting area near a window to be closer to natural light sources.
- Take breaks outdoors to soak up the sun and reset your internal clock.
- Consider installing light tubes or skylights to bring natural light into darker areas of your home.

7.2 The Power of Color: Influencing Mood and Energy Levels

Color has a significant influence on our mood, energy levels, and mental wellbeing. Enumerating a few tips to incorporate color to bolster your health:

- Choose relaxing colors such as blues, greens, and earth tones for bedrooms and other areas meant for relaxation.
- Utilize energizing colors, like reds and oranges, in spaces meant for activity or creativity, such as workout rooms or home offices.
- Experiment with different color combinations to find what works best for your personality, preferences, and desired outcomes.
- Consider using color therapy lamps or bulbs that emit a specific color to influence your mood and energy levels in different spaces.

7.3 Air Quality and Home Detoxification

Indoor air quality is critical for maintaining good health. Unfortunately, many homes have poor air quality due to allergens, pet dander, germs, and harmful chemicals emitted from furniture, paint, and cleaning products. Improve indoor air quality by:

- Ensuring proper ventilation and circulation of fresh air through your dwelling.
- Investing in high-quality air purifiers and HVAC filters for cleaning the air.
- Choosing non-toxic, eco-friendly cleaning and personal care products.
- Incorporating indoor plants that can help filter toxins and improve air quality.

7.4 Temperature Control for Optimal Sleep and Recovery

Our body's response to temperature plays a significant part in our sleep quality and recovery. Keeping our bedroom cool and comfortable can positively impact sleep duration and quality:

- Maintain an optimal bedroom temperature of around 60-67°F (15-19°C) for ideal sleeping conditions.
- Invest in temperature-regulating sheets, mattress toppers, and sleepwear made from moisture-wicking materials like bamboo and eucalyptus.
- Use blackout curtains or shades to block out any heat or light from outside.
- Experiment with thermostat settings to find your ideal sleep temperature.

7.5 Designing Spaces for Movement, Mindfulness, and Connection

Our environment can encourage healthy habits and behaviors such as regular physical activity, mindfulness practices, and social connections. Assess your living spaces and consider making these modifications:

- Create a designated workout area with easy access to fitness equipment and exercise materials.
- Carve out a peaceful, clutter-free zone for meditation, relaxation, or yoga.
- Set up comfortable seating arrangements for socializing with friends and family, fostering connection and support.
- Design your workspace ergonomically to promote good posture, minimize strain, and encourage short stretch breaks during your workday.

7.6 Decluttering and Organizing Your Space for Better Mental Health

Keeping our environment decluttered and organized can have a positive effect on our mental health and make it easier to maintain healthy habits. A few tips for creating an orderly space:

- Take the time to declutter your home by getting rid of extraneous items or unnecessary belongings.
- Invest in practical storage solutions to keep your space organized and clutter-free.
- Incorporate aesthetically pleasing décor that serves a purpose or brings joy, such as art or houseplants.
- Develop a routine for keeping your space clean and organized, making it easier to maintain a healthy environment.

In conclusion, by adopting these environmental adaptation strategies, you can dramatically improve your health, longevity, and overall well-being. Acknowledge the transformative potential of your surroundings, and take proactive steps to shape your living spaces into a launchpad for your journey towards optimal health.

7.1 The Health-Focused Home: Creating a Space That Boosts Longevity

As biohackers, we understand the significance of integrating various techniques and technologies that help streamline and optimize our physiological, mental, and emotional well-being. Most often, this journey goes beyond diet and exercise, delving into various facets of our lives—especially our living environment.

Our home environment plays a crucial role in our overall health, having potential implications on our sleep, stress, energy levels, and tendency to make positive decisions. As such, we should treat our homes as sanctuaries that nourish, recharge, and assist us in maximizing our longevity.

In this chapter, we'll explore the various elements of a health-focused home, along with actionable steps to modify your living space in favor of supporting longevity.

7.1.1 Air Quality: Breathe Easy for Longevity

Indoor air pollution is an often-overlooked threat to human health. Since we spend approximately 90% of our lives indoors, improving the quality of air in our living spaces should be a top priority for longevity biohackers.

- **Purify the air**: Invest in air purifiers that utilize HEPA filters, which can remove over 99% of airborne particles. Position these devices in your living areas and bedrooms. Ideally, you should also choose one with an activated carbon filter for optimal results.
- **Control humidity**: Excess moisture can encourage the growth of mold and other allergens. Aim to maintain an indoor humidity level of around 40 to 60% by using a dehumidifier or humidifier, as needed.
- **Introduce indoor plants**: Some houseplants are natural air purifiers, capable of removing volatile organic compounds (VOCs) and other toxins from the air. Spider plants, peace lilies, and snake plants are all effective choices.
- **Avoid toxic cleaning products**: Switch to eco-friendly household cleaners, or use natural alternatives like white vinegar and baking soda to minimize your exposure to harmful chemicals.

7.1.2 Water Quality: Quench Your Thirst with the Purest Drink

Having access to clean, contaminant-free water is vital for overall health and longevity.

- **Filter your water**: Investing in a high-quality water filtration system, or even a faucet-mounted filter, can help reduce contaminants, including heavy metals, bacteria, and other impurities. Reverse osmosis filters are a top choice for the most comprehensive filtration.
- **Store water wisely**: Avoid plastic containers, as these can leach harmful chemicals into your water. Instead, opt for glass, ceramic, or stainless-steel vessels.

7.1.3 Light Exposure: Using Light to Your Advantage

Optimizing your exposure to natural and artificial light is an integral part of supporting healthy sleep-wake patterns and overall well-being.

- **Embrace natural light**: Allow as much natural daylight into your living spaces as possible. Sunlight boosts vitamin D production and is vital for regulating our circadian rhythm.
- **Limit blue light exposure**: Exposure to blue light from screens, LEDs, and fluorescent lights can wreak havoc on our sleep and overall health. Target reducing your reliance on these sources during the evening. You can also use blue light filtering tools like screen protectors, glasses, or software to minimize the impact.
- **Leverage red light therapy**: Red and infrared light therapy can improve cellular health, promote

relaxation, and support recovery. Devices such as lamps, panels, or bulbs can be used to incorporate this biohack into your living space.

7.1.4 Space Organization: Creating an Orderly Environment

A clutter-free, organized environment helps to reduce stress, promote productivity, and optimize overall health.

- **Declutter**: Regularly evaluate your possessions and get rid of items that no longer serve a purpose. Adopt a minimalistic mindset, only keeping items that offer function or truly spark joy.
- **Designate functional zones**: Carve out specific areas in your home for different activities like work, exercise, relaxation, and sleeping. This will help to delineate spaces, creating optimal environments for each activity.

7.1.5 Sleep Sanctuary: Optimize Your Bedroom for Restful Slumber

Design your bedroom to promote restorative, deep sleep—a major tenet of health and longevity.

- **Dark and cool**: Your bedroom should be as dark as possible, utilizing blackout curtains and removing any sources of light. It should also be cool, with an ideal temperature of around 62-67°F (16-19°C).
- **Invest in quality**: Select a comfortable mattress, pillow, and bedding that enhance your sleep experience. Investing in these crucial elements pays off in both quality of rest and long-term health.

- **Free from distractions**: Keep electronic devices out of your bedroom if possible, especially screens that emit blue light.
- **Neutral colors**: Opt for a calming, neutral color palette in your bedroom to promote relaxation and signal your brain that it's time to rest.

By looking at your living space holistically and making intentional changes, you can create an environment that actively supports your well-being each day. The environmental adaptation is a key component in the biohacker's journey toward optimal health and longevity.

Environmental Adaptation: Shaping Your Space for Health and Longevity

In this chapter, we discuss how you can shape your environment to encourage optimal health and maximize longevity. Just as animals and plants have adapted to their environments to survive and thrive, we too can harness the power of environmental adaptation to nurture our bodies and minds. By understanding our ability to influence our surroundings, we can make purposeful choices that create an environment that supports our biohacking goals.

How Environments Influence Our Health and Habits

Our environment plays a significant role in shaping our habits, choices, and overall health. The spaces we inhabit, whether they are our homes, workplaces, or social settings, can dictate our behaviors and routine activities. In turn, these behaviors contribute to our daily nutrient intake, exercise routines, sleep patterns, stress levels, and much more.

Therefore, if we want to reach our optimal health and propel ourselves towards longevity, it is essential to become aware of how our environment is influencing us and take a proactive role in molding it to better match our biohacking objectives.

The Four Pillars of Environmental Adaptation

We can divide the process of environmental adaptation into four main pillars:

1. **Nutrition Adaptation:** Creating a dietary environment that aligns with our biohacking goals.
2. **Physical Activity Adaptation:** Designing spaces that encourage movement and exercise.
3. **Stress Reduction Adaptation:** Foster a stress-reducing environment to support mental health and well-being.
4. **Sleep Optimization Adaptation:** Establish a sleep-conducive living space to ensure quality slumber and restorative rest.

We will explore each of these pillars in greater detail below.

1. Nutrition Adaptation

Choosing the right foods is one of the foundational aspects of accomplishing optimal health. However, it can be difficult to make healthy dietary choices if our environment is filled with unhealthier options. Here are some ways you can adapt your environment to promote healthier eating habits:

- **Kitchen Layout:** Organize your kitchen in such a way that the healthier choices are more easily accessible. This might include placing healthy snacks on the most visible shelves and storing unhealthier options out of reach or sight.
- **Meal Preparation:** Set aside time to prepare healthy meals in advance, which will make it more likely that you make healthier choices when hunger strikes. This can also help reduce the chances of opting for fast food or unhealthy convenience items.
- **Grocery Shopping:** Plan your grocery shopping such that you buy only the items you need for your healthy meal plan. Avoid purchasing unhealthy, processed foods that do not align with your health goals. Stick to a list and resist the temptation to buy items out of impulse.
- **Social Eating:** It can be challenging to adhere to a healthy diet when those around you are indulging in unhealthy treats. Surround yourself with people who support your biohacking goals and participate in activities that involve healthier eating options.

2. Physical Activity Adaptation

Staying active is crucial for maintaining overall health and well-being. Here are some ways you can adapt your environment to inspire more movement and exercise:

- **Home Workout Space:** Designate a dedicated space in your home where you can perform exercise routines or practice yoga or stretching. Keep this area stocked with basic workout equipment such as resistance bands, kettlebells, and yoga mats.

- **Standing Desk:** Experiment with a standing or adjustable-height desk to reduce the amount of time you spend sitting each day. Sitting for extended periods is associated with poor health outcomes, so incorporating more standing or walking breaks can be beneficial.
- **Walkable Destinations:** Choose your living and working locations with walkability in mind. Aim to live in areas that provide access to parks, walking paths, and essential amenities within walking or cycling distance.
- **Social Activity:** Engage in physical activities with friends, family, and coworkers. Organize social events around activities such as hiking, cycling, or group fitness classes, which bring both physical and social benefits.

3. Stress Reduction Adaptation

Our environment can heavily influence our stress levels. Here are some strategies for creating a stress-reducing environment to support better mental health and longevity:

- **Green Spaces:** Incorporate plants and greenery into your living and working spaces. Research shows that green spaces have a calming effect and can help reduce stress levels.
- **Natural Light:** Ensure that your living and workspaces have access to plenty of natural light. Exposure to natural light during daylight hours has been linked with improved mood and cognitive function.
- **De-clutter:** Keep your surroundings organized and clutter-free. A messy environment can contribute to increased feelings of stress and overwhelm.

- **Relaxation Spaces:** Designate specific areas in your home or workspace that are reserved for relaxation and decompression. This can include a cozy reading nook or a dedicated space for meditation.

4. Sleep Optimization Adaptation

Quality sleep is crucial for overall health and longevity. Boost your sleep quality by adapting your environment in the following ways:

- **Bedroom Sanctuary:** Transform your bedroom into a restful sleep sanctuary by ensuring it is clean, clutter-free, and features a comfortable mattress and pillows. Additionally, consider using blackout curtains to block out unwanted light and sound.
- **Temperature Regulation:** Keep your bedroom temperature within the optimal range for sleep (approximately 60-67 degrees Fahrenheit). Experiment with different bedding materials and types, as well as sleepwear, to address your personal temperature preferences.
- **Electronics-free Zone:** Avoid using electronic devices such as smartphones, tablets, or laptops in the bedroom. The blue light emitted from these screens can disrupt the production of the sleep hormone melatonin, making it harder to fall asleep.
- **Wind-down Routine:** Cultivate a nightly wind-down routine that helps signal to your mind and body that it's time for rest. This might include reading, practicing gentle stretches or yoga, or participating in a short meditation session.

By understanding the profound impact our environment has on our overall health and longevity, we can take an active stance in shaping it to better align with our biohacking objectives. Experiment with different strategies within each of the four pillars of adaptation and customize your surroundings to support your journey towards optimal health and enhanced longevity.

8. Upgrading Biomechanics: Optimizing Movement and Posture

8.1 Understanding Your Body's Architecture

8.1.1 The Skeletal System

Before diving into the intricacies of optimizing movement and posture, it is essential to have a basic understanding of the human body's architecture. At the core of this architecture lies the skeletal system. Comprised of 206 bones, the skeleton provides structural support and protection for internal organs, enables movement by serving as attachment points for muscles, and plays a role in mineral storage and hematopoiesis (the formation of blood cellular components).

Bones can be categorized into four types: long bones (such as the femur, tibia, and fibula), short bones (such as the bones in the wrists and ankles), flat bones (such as the sternum and skull), and irregular bones (such as the vertebrae). Each bone is designed to provide particular mechanical advantages that determine how they fit together and interact with surrounding muscles, tendons, and ligaments.

8.1.2 The Muscular System

The muscular system is comprised of over 600 muscles responsible for the various actions and forces associated with movement. Skeletal muscles contract to create tension, pulling on bones to produce movement at a joint. Much like the bones, muscles are organized into groups based on their location, function, and mechanical advantage.

Muscles can be arranged in several different ways: parallel (running in the same direction); convergent (narrowing towards a single attachment point); pennate (feather-like arrangement); and circular (forming a ring around an opening). Each arrangement is designed to optimize force production, speed, and range of motion for specific actions.

8.1.3 Joints and Movement

Joints are where two or more bones meet, allowing for a range of motion between them. Some joints permit a vast range of motion, such as the ball-and-socket joints (like the hip joint), while others provide more stability with minimal movement, like the hinge joint at the elbow. The trade-off between mobility and stability is a critical factor in maintaining overall joint health and preventing injury.

Joint movement can be classified into several types: flexion (bending); extension (straightening); abduction (movement away from the midline); adduction (movement towards the midline); and rotation (movement around a single axis). Understanding these movements and their associated ranges of motion is vital when seeking to optimize biomechanics and reduce the risk of injury.

8.1.4 Connective Tissue and Stability

For bones and muscles to work together effectively, they rely on a complex network of connective tissues, including tendons, ligaments, and fascia. Tendons attach muscle to bones, allowing for the transmission of forces necessary for movement. Ligaments connect bones to other bones, providing stability and support for joints. Fascia is a continuous network of connective tissue that surrounds muscles, providing structural support while allowing for sliding and gliding between adjacent structures.

8.2 Assessing Your Movement and Posture

8.2.1 Postural Assessment

Having a thorough understanding of your body's natural alignment can offer valuable insights into potential areas of concern or weakness. This knowledge can then be used to develop targeted strategies for optimizing posture and mitigating the risk of injury. Postural assessments can be as simple as observing oneself in a full-length mirror or as advanced as using specialized software to analyze gait, muscle imbalances, and other biomechanical factors.

Key areas to consider during a postural assessment include head and neck alignment, shoulder positioning, spinal curvature, hip alignment, and weight distribution through the feet. Be aware of any deviations from proper alignment and symmetry, as these may indicate areas in need of further attention or strengthening.

8.2.2 Functional Movement Screening

A functional movement screen (FMS) is another valuable tool in assessing biomechanics, providing a comprehensive analysis of movement patterns and identifying any dysfunctions that might be present. The FMS typically involves a series of exercises designed to test flexibility, mobility, and stability across various joints and muscles. These exercises may reveal asymmetries, limitations, or compensations that can inform targeted interventions to improve movement quality.

8.3 Strategies for Optimizing Movement and Posture

8.3.1 Strengthening Weak Muscles

Muscle imbalances can have a significant impact on biomechanical efficiency and postural alignment. By identifying and targeting weak or underactive muscles, it is possible to improve overall stability and movement efficiency, potentially reducing the risk of injury.

8.3.2 Stretching and Mobility Work

Incorporating a mix of stretching and mobility exercises into your daily routine can help to improve joint range of motion, ensuring that muscles and connective tissues remain supple and elastic. This, in turn, can result in better movement mechanics and overall body function.

8.3.3 Posture Qualities and Ergonomics

Being conscious of your posture and positioning throughout the day—particularly during activities that require prolonged periods of sitting or standing—is crucial in maintaining optimal alignment and preventing postural deviations. Ergonomics plays a significant role in achieving good posture, so consider refining your workspace, chair, and bed to support your body's natural curvature and positioning.

Increasing your awareness of how your body moves through space can provide valuable insights into any biomechanical dysfunctions or habits that may be impacting your overall movement and posture. Practice engaging your senses while performing everyday tasks or exercise, and pay close attention to how your body responds to different stimuli. This awareness can lead to more efficient patterns of movement and a greater sense of control over your biomechanics.

By incorporating these concepts and strategies into your daily routine, you're well on your way to achieving optimal biomechanical efficiency, improved posture, and a more robust foundation for overall health and well-being.

Maximizing Mobility: Techniques to Enhance Your Flexibility and Stability

In the pursuit of optimal health, the importance of mobility cannot be overstated. As biohackers, we strive to optimize the intricate systems that our body relies on for optimal functioning. Mobility, which refers to the total movement capacity of joints and muscles, is a key aspect of our biomechanical functioning. Poor mobility can lead to discomfort, pain, injury, and reduced performance in daily activities or exercise routines. By upgrading our mobility, we can achieve better movement patterns, improved biomechanics, and maintain lifelong joint and muscular health.

Understanding Mobility: Range of Motion, Flexibility, and Stability

Mobility is a complex aspect of biomechanics, encompassing the range of motion (ROM) available at a joint, the flexibility of the muscles and connective tissues surrounding that joint, and the stability provided by the ligamentous and muscular structures which support the joint. Upgrading our mobility requires interventions that target each of these components, while recognizing that a balance between ROM, flexibility, and stability is essential for the prevention of injuries, optimization of movement patterns, and maintenance of a healthy musculoskeletal system.

Assessing your Mobility: Evaluating Your Starting Point

Before attempting to improve your mobility, it's important to get a clear picture of your existing movement patterns and flexibility. There are several baseline mobility assessments available that can serve as benchmarks to track your progress over time. Some of these assessments include functional movement screens, range of motion testing, and posture evaluations. Conducting these assessments regularly will help you identify strengths, weaknesses, and any imbalances in your mobility, allowing you to create a targeted biohacking plan specifically for your needs.

The Mobility Toolbox: Techniques and Tools to Enhance Your Biomechanics

1. **Dynamic Stretching and Warm-Ups:** Before engaging in any kind of physical activity or exercise, taking the time for an appropriate warm-up is essential. Dynamic stretching, as opposed to static, involves active movements that take the muscles through a full range of motion without holding any position for an extended period. This type of

stretching activates muscle tissue, increases blood flow, lubricates joints, and prepares the nervous system for higher levels of activity.

2. **Static and Assisted Stretching:** Static stretching is the act of holding a stretch for an extended period (15-30 seconds) without bouncing. While it should not be confused with a warm-up, it can play an essential role in developing flexibility over time. Static stretching should be performed post-exercise or as a stand-alone practice to help increase muscle length and tissue mobility. Assisted stretching, on the other hand, enlists the help of a partner or a device (like a resistance band or yoga strap) to help deepen the stretch.

3. **Self-Myofascial Release (SMR):** SMR, using tools like foam rollers or massage balls, can be used to target specific areas of tightness or discomfort by applying pressure and slow movements. It aids in releasing restrictions and adhesions in the muscle and surrounding fascia, reducing tension and increasing flexibility.

4. **Strength Training for Stability:** Targeted strength training exercises that emphasize stabilizing muscles (particularly surrounding the core, shoulders, and hips) can greatly improve joint stability and therefore overall mobility. Functional strength exercises, like single-leg balance work or stability ball exercises, can be especially beneficial.

5. **Yoga and Pilates:** These mind-body practices combine elements of stretching, core strengthening, and breath control to increase flexibility, stability, and overall muscle control. Incorporating regular yoga or Pilates practice into your routine can lead to significant improvements in mobility over time.

6. **Mobilization Techniques:** Joint mobilizations, such as those performed by physical therapists and

chiropractors, involve precise, targeted movements to help restore joint movement and reduce pain. Educating yourself about effective mobilization techniques can be beneficial for on-the-spot self-treatment or as a long-term preventive strategy.

7. **Consistency and Patience:** Just as building strength or losing weight takes time and consistency, so too does improving mobility. Patience and a commitment to a consistent practice, using the tools and techniques described above, will yield the best results in the long term.

Monitoring Progress and Constant Adjustment

As with all biohacking pursuits, monitoring progress and making adjustments to your mobility plan is key to achieving optimal results. Regularly reassess your mobility using the assessments mentioned earlier, and be prepared to modify your practice as your needs change. Remember that improved mobility will support your overall biomechanical functioning, allowing you to perform better, experience less pain, and maintain a healthy body for years to come.

8.1 Understanding Body Mechanics: The Foundation for Optimal Movement and Posture

Before diving into the methods for optimizing movement and posture, it's essential to first understand the basics of body mechanics. Body mechanics refers to the way our bodies move and maintain balance while performing various physical activities. Good body mechanics reduces strain on the muscles, joints, and spine, helping to prevent injuries and increase overall health and efficiency. Furthermore, when our biomechanics are operating optimally, it allows us to perform tasks with greater ease and maintain comfort throughout the day.

8.1.1 The Building Blocks: Bones, Joints, Muscles, and Tendons

To understand body mechanics, we need to first look at the main components responsible for movement and posture: bones, joints, muscles, and tendons. The human skeletal system consists of approximately 206 bones, which serve as the framework for our body. These bones are connected by joints, which allow for movement and provide mechanical support. Muscles, on the other hand, are responsible for creating motion by contracting and relaxing. Finally, tendons are the fibrous tissues that connect muscles to bones, allowing them to exert force on the skeleton during movement.

8.1.2 Proper Alignment: The Key to Good Body Mechanics

One of the essential aspects of good body mechanics is maintaining proper alignment throughout various postures and movements. In a neutral posture, the ears, shoulders, hips, knees, and ankles should all be aligned in a straight line. Proper alignment promotes better balance, reduces strain on muscles and joints, and allows our body to function more efficiently, ultimately resulting in less pain and discomfort.

Here are some key points to remember for maintaining proper alignment:

- Keep your head up, looking forward rather than down.

- Keep your shoulders back and relaxed.
- Maintain a slight curve in your lower back, but avoid overarching.
- Engage your abdominal muscles to provide additional support to your spine.
- Make sure your hips are level, with one slightly above the other.
- Keep your knees slightly bent, avoiding locking them out.
- Maintain an even distribution of weight between your feet.

8.1.3 The Importance of Ergonomics and Body Awareness

Ergonomics is the practice of designing our environment according to our body's needs and limitations, helping us perform tasks more efficiently, while minimizing discomfort and risk of injury. This includes the design of our workstations, chairs, tools, and even our mobile devices. By adapting our environment to fit our biomechanical needs, we reduce the strain on our body, helping to promote better posture, movement, and overall health.

Body awareness is another crucial component for achieving optimal biomechanics. Developing an awareness of how our body feels and moves allows us to recognize when we are out of alignment, placing unnecessary stress on our muscles and joints. By becoming more conscious of our body's movements and sensations, we can make corrections in real-time, preventing potential injuries, and promoting better posture and overall well-being.

8.1.4 Incorporating Exercise and Movement for Optimal Body Mechanics

Regular physical activity, including strength training, stretching, and aerobic exercises, is essential for maintaining good body mechanics. Strength training helps build the muscles necessary to support proper alignment and prevent injury, while stretching helps improve flexibility and range of motion. Aerobic exercises, such as walking, running, swimming, or cycling, help build stamina, promote circulation, and improve overall cardiovascular health.

Movement also plays a vital role in promoting optimal body mechanics. By integrating regular movement throughout the day, we can counteract the negative effects of prolonged sitting, such as muscle weakness, joint stiffness, and poor posture. Aim to take short breaks every hour, even if it's as simple as standing up and stretching or going for a brief walk.

8.1.5 Additional Techniques for Optimizing Body Mechanics

In addition to the points mentioned above, there are several other techniques that can contribute to optimizing your body mechanics. Some of these include:

- Understand your body's limits: While pushing ourselves physically can be beneficial, it's essential to recognize our body's limitations to avoid potential injuries. Know when to stop or modify an activity to prevent strain on your muscles and joints.
- Warm-up and cool-down: Incorporating a thorough warm-up and cool-down period before and after exercise reduces the risk of injury and prepares our muscles and joints for the activity.
- Practice good form: Whether lifting weights, running, or simply walking, it's crucial to prioritize proper form

and technique to protect and promote our body's biomechanics.

- Utilize supportive footwear: Depending on the activity, support and cushioning in shoes can provide stability, helping to maintain proper alignment and balance.
- Seek professional guidance: A physical therapist or certified personal trainer can help assess your body mechanics and provide recommendations to improve your posture, alignment, and movement patterns.

In conclusion, optimizing our body mechanics through proper alignment, ergonomics, body awareness, exercise, and additional techniques can significantly enhance our overall health and well-being. By mastering the foundations of biomechanics, we empower ourselves to move more efficiently, reduce the risk of injury, and experience greater comfort and ease in our daily lives. Remember, our bodies are designed for movement, and it's our responsibility to ensure that they function optimally by prioritizing good body mechanics.

8.1 Mastering the Musculoskeletal System: Building a Better Foundation

Before we delve into the complex world of biomechanics and the innovative ways to optimize our movements and posture, it is essential to understand the fundamental structure that supports our every motion - the musculoskeletal system. Comprising bones, muscles, tendons, ligaments, and other supporting tissues, the musculoskeletal system is the foundation for all physical activity. Strengthening and maintaining this system is the first step towards enhancing biomechanics and improving overall health.

8.1.1 Musculoskeletal System 101: Bones, Muscles, and Connective Tissues

The musculoskeletal system is composed of several key components that, when working in harmony, allow us to function optimally. The primary elements of this system include:

- **Bones**: Rigid and strong, bones act as the framework for our bodies, providing support and structure. The human skeleton consists of 206 bones, which are connected by flexible joints that provide a range of motion. Bones also serve as a mineral reservoir, housing essential nutrients like calcium and phosphorus.
- **Muscles**: Comprising roughly 40-45% of our body mass, muscles are the primary drivers of movement. They work in pairs or groups to contract and expand, generating force to move bones at their respective joints. Muscles also play a crucial role in stabilizing joints and maintaining posture.
- **Tendons**: These bands of fibrous connective tissue attach muscles to bones, ensuring proper joint function and movement. Tendons are strong yet somewhat flexible, allowing for efficient force transfer from muscles to bones.
- **Ligaments**: Much like tendons, ligaments are bands of fibrous connective tissue, but they serve to connect bones to each other, providing stability and integrity to joints.
- **Cartilage**: This smooth, flexible connective tissue provides cushioning between bones and enables joint surfaces to glide smoothly against each other. It also serves as structural support in various parts of our bodies, such as our ears and nose.

Understanding these fundamental elements is key in safeguarding and enhancing the functioning of our musculoskeletal system.

8.1.2 Biomechanical Optimization: Balancing Strength, Flexibility, and Stability

In order to optimize movement and posture, we need to strike a balance between the complementary components of the musculoskeletal system: strength, flexibility, and stability.

- **Strength**: Utilizing a mix of resistance training and functional movements, increasing muscular strength not only primes our bodies for greater physical activity, but it can also help protect against injuries and reduce the risk of certain conditions such as sarcopenia (age-related muscle loss).
- **Flexibility**: Maintaining an adequate range of motion is crucial for optimal biomechanics. A combination of static and dynamic stretching, as well as practices such as yoga or Pilates, can help improve flexibility and promote better posture, reducing the risk of injury and enhancing overall functionality.
- **Stability**: Ensuring joint stability and balance is vital in all aspects of biomechanics. Core strengthening exercises and balance training, such as incorporating stability balls or BOSU® trainers into your routine, can help provide a solid foundation for efficient movement and reduce the risk of falls or injuries.

8.1.3 Posture: Alignment for Optimal Performance

Our posture - the way we align our bodies while sitting, standing, or moving - has a significant impact on our biomechanics, potentially influencing everything from athletic performance to musculoskeletal health.

Poor posture can lead to a variety of issues, including muscle imbalances, joint stress, reduced vital capacity, and even impeded digestion. In contrast, maintaining a neutral spine position with properly aligned shoulders, hips, and knees allows for efficient movement and reduced stress on the musculoskeletal system.

To improve posture, consider employing a mix of exercises that target postural muscles (such as those found in the core and upper back), as well as regular posture checks and adjustments throughout the day. Additionally, optimizing your workspace and sleeping conditions for better alignment can also help improve your overall posture.

8.1.4 Injury Prevention & Recovery: Prioritizing Healing and Growth

No matter how well we optimize our movements and posture, injuries can still occur. Understanding how to properly recover from and rehabilitate these injuries is just as important as taking steps to prevent them.

- **Rest**: Upon experiencing an injury, the initial stage of rehabilitation involves rest, allowing our bodies to begin the healing process.
- **Ice, Compression, Elevation, & Immobilization**: Applying Ice to reduce swelling, utilizing compression to stabilize injured areas, elevating injured limbs for proper blood flow, and immobilizing the affected area with splints or casts are essential steps in the early recovery process.
- **Physical Therapy & Rehabilitation**: As the injury begins to heal, working with a qualified physical

therapist to progressively reintroduce activity, strength exercises, and stretching can help restore function and prevent future injuries.
- **Preventative Measures**: Understanding and addressing the root cause of an injury, such as insufficient warm-up, muscle imbalances, or overtraining, can help reduce the risk of future injury recurrence.

By respecting our bodies and taking the necessary steps to prevent and rehabilitate injuries, we lay the groundwork for optimized biomechanics and long-term health.

In conclusion, the road to upgrading biomechanics starts with understanding and maintaining a healthy musculoskeletal system, striving for a harmonious balance of strength, flexibility, and stability, as well as practicing proper posture and prioritizing injury prevention and recovery. By optimizing these foundational elements within our bodies, we pave the way for enhanced athletic performance, greater overall health, and longevity.

Biomechanics 101: The Foundation of Optimal Movement and Posture

Before diving into specific strategies and techniques you can use to upgrade your biomechanics, it's important to build a foundation of understanding. This includes learning about the basic principles of biomechanics and how these principles apply to the body's movement and posture.

A. The Basics of Biomechanics

Biomechanics is the study of the forces acting upon and within biological structures, as well as the effects these forces produce on living organisms. It combines principles from both physics and biology to analyze the mechanical aspects of movement and posture. Here are a few fundamental principles you need to know:

1. **Force:** A push or pull exerted on an object, including biological structures. Forces are responsible for changing an object's state of motion or its shape - this also applies to your body.
2. **Equilibrium:** When forces acting on an object are balanced, leaving the object in a state of rest or constant velocity. The human body is constantly working to maintain a state of equilibrium and, as you'll see, optimizing movement and posture helps maintain this state.
3. **Lever Systems:** Levers consist of a rigid bar (like a bone) that rotates around a fixed point called a fulcrum (usually a joint). Muscles pulling on bones create the force necessary for human movement. Levers allow for force to be applied effectively and efficiently.
4. **Tensile and Compressive Forces:** Tensile forces involve pulling and stretching, while compressive forces involve pushing and shortening. For example, when jumping, leg extension is enabled by compressive forces in the bones and tensile forces in the muscles.
5. **Stability:** **To maintain balance and support during movement, the body employs stability from muscles and bones. The greater the stability, the less likely the body is to be injured or imbalanced during motion.

B. Anatomy and Biomechanics

Understanding the biomechanics of human movement and posture requires some knowledge of anatomy. The body consists of various systems that all contribute to your ability to move and maintain proper posture:

1. **Musculoskeletal System:** This system is composed of your muscles and bones, and is responsible for the body's stability, support, and movement. Your muscles generate force and motion, while your bones provide structure and leverage.
2. **Nervous System:** The nervous system sends signals between the brain and the rest of the body, controlling movement and coordination. Good biomechanics depend on effective communication between these two systems.
3. **Articular System:** This system consists of your body's joints, which connect your bones and allow for movement. Healthy joint function is essential for optimal movement and posture.

C. Assessing and Addressing Posture and Movement Dysfunction

Proper alignment and function of the spine and joints are critical for good posture and movement. The most common causes of poor posture and movement dysfunction are muscular imbalances, joint misalignments, and biomechanical inefficiencies. Performing a simple self-assessment can help you identify and address these issues:

1. Evaluate your posture: Stand in front of a mirror and check for rounded shoulders, a forward head, uneven hips, crooked spine, or other irregularities.
2. Assess muscle imbalances: Pay attention to any muscles that may be tight, weak, or overworked. Common problem areas include the chest, upper back, neck, hips, and lower back.

3. Identify joint misalignments: Take note of any joints that may be limited in mobility, such as restricted ankle dorsiflexion or limited hip extension.
4. Evaluate biomechanical inefficiencies: Take note of any movement patterns that may be inefficient or incorrect. For example, do your knees cave in during a squat, or do you hunch your back when bending over?

Once you've identified these problem areas, you can take action to address them. This may involve targeted mobility work, strengthening exercises, or improvements in movement technique – all of which will contribute to better biomechanics and overall health.

Strategies for Upgrading Biomechanics

Now that you have a foundational understanding of biomechanics and how they relate to posture and movement, let's explore some strategies for optimizing your own biomechanics:

1. **Mobility and Flexibility:** Improving and maintaining mobility and flexibility enables your joints to function at their full range of motion, which in turn helps establish proper biomechanics. Incorporate regular stretching and mobility exercises into your routine, targeting all major muscle groups.
2. **Strength and Stability Training:** Strengthening the muscles that support proper biomechanics can help you maintain better posture and movement patterns. Focus on exercises that target the core and posture muscles, as well as compound movements that engage multiple muscle groups and joints.

3. **Technique and Skill Development:** Developing proper technique in all movements, from everyday activities to exercise, is crucial for establishing efficient and safe biomechanics. Practicing functional movement patterns, like squatting, hinging, lunging, pushing, and pulling, with a focus on precision and form, can help improve technique and biomechanical efficiency.
4. **Posture Awareness and Correction:** Building an awareness of your posture throughout the day is key to maintaining good biomechanics. Make a conscious effort to correct any postural abnormalities you notice, whether sitting, standing, or moving.
5. **Ergonomic Adjustments:** Ensuring your work and living environment supports proper posture and biomechanics can have a significant impact on your overall health. Adjust your desk setup, seating, and other aspects of your environment to promote good posture and reduce strain on the body.

With a better understanding of biomechanics and the actionable strategies above, you can enhance your body's function, reduce the risk of injury, and promote overall health and well-being. Optimal movement and posture will serve as a foundation for your biohacking journey, allowing you to perform at your best in all aspects of life.

9. Cutting-Edge Technologies: Enhancing the Body from the Inside Out

9.3 Nanotechnology: The Future of Biohacking

Nanotechnology, the branch of technology that deals with molecular-scale precision, has the potential to revolutionize the field of biohacking by enabling precise manipulation of the human body and enhancing performance through internal adjustments. Applications of nanotechnology in medicine, commonly known as nanomedicine, usually focus on innovative drug delivery systems and advanced imaging agents, but the use of nanoscale devices to enhance human abilities, often referred to as nanocyborgs, is a fascinating domain of research that could lead to a whole new era of human enhancement. In this subsection, we will explore some of the breakthroughs in nanotechnology that could have significant implications in the field of biohacking.

9.3.1 Nano-Sensors: Monitoring Health at the Molecular Level

One of the most promising applications of nano-scale devices in the world of biohacking is the development of nano-sensors — tiny particles which can be incorporated into the human body to monitor important biological processes. These nano-sensors can be fashioned to detect specific molecules or cellular byproducts, such as biomarkers for inflammation, infection, or chronic diseases.

Nano-sensors in the bloodstream could revolutionize healthcare by providing constant monitoring of biomarkers and other indicators for health. This continuous real-time feedback could help individuals make more informed choices about their habits, nutrition, and lifestyle practices, ultimately helping them to optimize their health and overall mental and physical performance.

9.3.2 Nano-Enhancement: The Next Frontier for Physical and Cognitive Abilities

Another domain of nanotechnology that may drastically impact biohacking is the enhancement of our physical and mental abilities through the use of nano-scale devices. This could be achieved through a variety of methods, including nano-scale implants, nanobots, and even the engineering of cell structures.

- **Nano-Implants**: These sub-microscopic implantable devices could be used to stimulate nerve cells, trigger the release of neurotransmitters, or even adjust the brain's electrical activity. This could lead to improvements in memory, cognitive speed, and a whole host of other neurological improvements. On the physical side, nano-implants could be used to stimulate muscles, alter pain perception, and even transform physical sensations such as touch.
- **Nanobots**: Nanorobots or nanobots are microscopic robots that could have far-reaching implications in the field of biohacking. Nanobots have been proposed to provide a range of enhancements, such as optimizing immune function by identifying and attacking foreign invaders swiftly, or targeting and repairing damaged cells or tissue at the molecular level.
- **Cellular Engineering**: Although still a distant reality, some biohackers propose the use of nano-scale devices to manipulate cellular or genetic structures within the body. This could, in theory, allow individuals to modify or introduce new genes to produce desirable attributes, such as faster processing speed

or the ability to see in different parts of the electromagnetic spectrum, as some animals can do.

9.3.3 The Ethical and Social Implications of Nanotechnology-Based Biohacking

While the potential applications of nanotechnology in biohacking are undeniably exciting, they also raise a plethora of ethical, moral, and social concerns that cannot go unaddressed. Access to advanced nanotechnology, especially for enhancement purposes, is likely to be costly, leading to a greater divide between the "haves" and "have-nots." Furthermore, issues of privacy and surveillance arise when considering the constant monitoring of our biological information that could be harvested by implanted nano-sensors.

Moreover, the possibility of individuals harnessing nano-scale devices to gain an unfair advantage over others could lead to social tensions and debates over whether to regulate, limit or ban the use of these technologies in specific domains, like sports or professional environments. As biohackers continue to push the boundaries of human enhancement, a fair and responsible approach to integrating new technologies will be required to maximize the benefits while minimizing potential adverse consequences.

Conclusion

Nanotechnology is poised to make a significant impact on the biohacking movement in the coming years. As nano-sensors, nano-enhancements, and various other applications of nanomedicine become more refined and accessible, the opportunities for individuals to optimize their health and performance will further expand. However, these technologies also introduce a myriad of ethical and social challenges that will need to be thoroughly explored and addressed in order to support equitable access and responsible usage. By considering the implications of emerging technologies, biohackers can harness the true potential of nanotechnology to advance human performance in a sustainable and ethical manner.

9.1. Bioelectronic Implants: The Convergence of Biology and Technology

In a world where technology constantly evolves to meet our needs more efficiently and health stands as our primary concern, the combination of biology and technology has given rise to bioelectronic implants. These innovative devices are designed to enhance the body's performance from the inside out and help monitor, treat or manage various health conditions. In this section, we will explore some of the most recent advancements in bioelectronic implants and their potential applications in biohacking for optimal health.

9.1.1. What are Bioelectronic Implants?

Bioelectronic implants are small, sophisticated devices that are embedded into the body to interact directly with our biological systems. They generally work by monitoring physiological data, stimulating specific nerves or muscles, or delivering targeted therapies. Some of the prominent examples of bioelectronic implants include cochlear implants for hearing restoration, retinal implants for vision restoration, deep brain stimulators for Parkinson's disease, and spinal cord stimulators for pain management.

9.1.2. The Key to Unlocking the Body's Communication Network

The endogenous electrical potential of the human body is the key to unlocking the therapeutic potential of bioelectronic implants. Our nervous system operates as a vast communication network, with electrical impulses transmitting signals between the brain and various organs or muscles. By decoding and modulating these signals, bioelectronic implants can deliver personalized therapy or control specific bodily functions, allowing for real-time monitoring, precise interventions, and exceptional outcomes.

9.1.3. Advancements in Bioelectronics Research

Recent developments in materials science, nanotechnology, and wireless communication have paved the way for groundbreaking research in bioelectronics. These advancements have resulted in more efficient, durable, and customizable bioelectronic implants, with the potential to revolutionize the way we perceive and manage health.

1. **Flexible and Stretchable Electronics**: With the advent of flexible and stretchable electronics, bioelectronic implants can now conform to the body's varied and dynamic surfaces. This has significantly increased the level of biocompatibility and reduced the risk of rejection, inflammation, or discomfort.
2. **Nanomaterials and Biodegradable Substrates**: The use of nanomaterials and biodegradable substrates has enabled miniaturization of bioelectronic implants to a size that can be safely and noninvasively inserted into the body. Moreover, the transient nature of these materials ensures that they degrade after the intended therapeutic period, avoiding long-term side effects or complications.

3. **Wireless Communication and Energy Harvesting**:
   The integration of wireless communication and energy
   harvesting techniques in bioelectronic implants has
   allowed for remote monitoring and adjusting of device
   settings, making the technology more user-friendly
   and adaptable.

9.1.4. Bioelectronic Implants and Biohacking

The use of bioelectronic implants can be seen as a form of
biohacking, where individuals take control of their own
biology to achieve optimal health. Some of the potential
applications of bioelectronic implants in biohacking include:

1. **Chronic Disease Management**: For individuals
   suffering from chronic diseases such as diabetes or
   hypertension, bioelectronic implants could serve as a
   means to monitor and regulate vital physiological
   parameters continuously. This can lead to more
   effective treatment and a better quality of life.
2. **Cognitive Enhancement**: Researchers are exploring
   the use of bioelectronic implants for memory
   augmentation, accelerated learning, and improved
   focus. By selectively modulating neural activity, these
   implants could unlock the full potential of the human
   brain.
3. **Physical Enhancement**: Bioelectronic implants can
   stimulate specific nerves or muscles to optimize
   physical performance, such as increasing endurance,
   speed, or strength. Athletes and fitness enthusiasts
   can benefit from this technology to surpass their
   biological limits.
4. **Sensory Augmentation**: Implants can also be used
   to enhance or restore sensory capabilities, such as
   vision or hearing. This technology can potentially
   benefit people suffering from sensory impairments, as

well as those seeking to expand their perceptual
range.

9.1.5. The Ethics of Bioelectronic Implants

As with any innovative technology, bioelectronic implants
raise concerns about ethics, privacy, and accessibility. Some
of the ethical questions surrounding this technology include:

1. **Therapeutic vs. Enhancement Uses**: The boundary
   between therapeutic and enhancement applications
   for bioelectronic implants can be blurry. While the
   primary goal of therapy is to restore normal function,
   enhancement seeks to surpass that level. There is a
   debate over whether society should endorse or limit
   the use of bioelectronics for non-medical purposes.
2. **Privacy and Data Security**: As bioelectronic implants
   are capable of wirelessly transmitting sensitive and
   personal health data, privacy and data security
   become crucial concerns. Ensuring data encryption
   and authorized access to this information is essential
   to protect individuals' rights.
3. **Access and Equity**: Ensuring that these cutting-edge
   technologies are accessible to everyone and not just
   limited to the privileged few is of paramount
   importance. Reducing the cost of bioelectronic
   implants, along with equitable distribution and
   availability, can ensure that their benefits are shared
   by all.

In conclusion, bioelectronic implants provide an exciting
opportunity to enhance the human body from the inside out
by tapping into our internal communication network. As
biohackers, understanding these technologies and their
potential impact on our health is essential to optimize our
innate biological potential fully. However, it is critical to weigh

the ethical implications and ensure the responsible use and equitable distribution of these powerful devices.

9.1 Nanotechnology: A New Frontier in Health Optimization

Nanotechnology plays a vital role in developing our understanding of the human body at a cellular and molecular level. Nanotechnology is proving itself indispensable in the quest to push the limits of our physical and mental potential, as biohackers look for new ways to enhance athletic performance, increase longevity, and improve overall health. In this section, we will discuss the different ways in which nanotechnology is changing our approach to achieving optimal health and how these advancements directly benefit our biohacking goals.

9.1.1 The Promise of Nanomedicine

Nanomedicine refers to the application of nanoscale technologies, such as nanoparticles and nanorobots, to diagnose, treat, and prevent diseases. The ability to manipulate atoms and molecules has yielded some exciting advancements in medicine, many of which are, or will be, crucial in treating conditions that were previously difficult or impossible to treat.

Some promising applications of nanomedicine include targeted drug delivery, disease detection and diagnosis, tissue repair, and gene therapy. Additionally, nanotechnology is instrumental in the development of personalized medicine, allowing medical professionals to tailor healthcare plans to each individual's unique genetic makeup and biochemical profile.

9.1.2 Targeted Drug Delivery: Superior Medication Efficiency

One of the most promising aspects of nanotechnology in medicine is targeted drug delivery. By encapsulating drug molecules within nanoparticles, it's possible to deliver them more efficiently to the specific cells and tissues in need of treatment. This targeted approach not only increases the therapeutic potential of the medication but also minimizes its adverse effects on the body.

In the realm of biohacking, targeted drug delivery could be used to enhance athletic performance, improve nutrient and supplement absorption, and maximize the effect of nootropics—cognitive-enhancing substances—on the brain, making it a cornerstone of the biohacker's toolkit.

9.1.3 Early Disease Detection and Diagnosis: Prevention Is Better Than Cure

Thanks to nanotechnology, disease detection is becoming more sensitive and less invasive. Nanoparticles are now being designed to identify molecular biomarkers that indicate the presence of diseases like cancer or Alzheimer's even before symptoms appear. Some nanoparticles can also be functionalized with imaging agents, allowing medical professionals to monitor the early stages of disease precisely and non-invasively.

Early detection and diagnosis are crucial components of biohacking's preventive approach to maximizing health and longevity. By catching diseases in their infancy, it becomes possible to promptly initiate personalized treatment plans and monitor their efficacy.

9.1.4 Tissue Repair and Regeneration: The Future of Healing

On the cutting edge of nanotechnology are nano-robots, also known as nanobots. These tiny devices, which can be programmed to carry out specific tasks within the body, hold significant potential for advanced biohacking.

One exciting application of nanobots is tissue repair and regeneration. By manipulating proteins and other biomolecules at a molecular level, nanobots could be used to repair damaged tissues from within the body, promoting accelerated healing. These tiny agents could also be programmed to stimulate cellular regeneration and rejuvenation, playing a vital role in achieving optimal health and wellness.

9.1.5 Gene Therapy: Tailoring the Human Genome

Another aspect of nanotechnology that has massive implications for biohacking is gene therapy. By delivering genetic material directly to cells, nanotechnology can create a new wave of therapeutic interventions that target the root causes of genetic diseases, slow aging, and even enhance human abilities.

For biohackers, gene therapy represents the ultimate frontier of self-improvement as it allows for the manipulation of the very building blocks of life. In the future, biohackers could use nanotechnology-enhanced gene therapy to optimize their body's functions, turning off or repairing genetic mutations responsible for diseases and aging while activating genes that boost performance, intelligence, and longevity.

9.1.6 Conclusion

Nanotechnology is redefining the frontiers of medicine, enabling revolutionary approaches to diagnosis, treatment, and prevention of diseases. As a core pillar of biohacking, nanotechnology provides biohackers with new tools and possibilities to achieve optimal health, both in preventing and treating diseases and in enhancing our innate abilities. While ethical and regulatory debates around nanotechnology continue, there's no doubt that this rapidly evolving field will have a lasting impact on the future of biohacking and our understanding of the human body.

9.1 Nanotechnology: Upgrading the Human Body at the Cellular Level

Considered a revolution in science and technology, nanotechnology is the manipulation of matter on an atomic, molecular, and supramolecular scale. It is a rapidly evolving field that is bridging disciplines, industries, and nations. At the forefront of this innovation lies the potential to transform biotechnology, especially in regards to human enhancement. Biohackers all over the world are excited about the opportunities nanotechnology may present to progress the human body beyond its natural limitations.

9.1.1 What is Nanotechnology?

Nanotechnology is the science, engineering, and application of functional systems at the nanometer scale: generally, systems with components smaller than 100 nanometers in size. This allows for the precise manipulation of molecules and atoms to create new materials, devices, and even new forms of life.

9.1.2 How Does Nanotechnology Apply to Biohacking?

By developing targeted applications at the cellular level, the field of nanotechnology is poised to make significant advancements in biotechnology. A biohacker's goal is to optimize the body's performance and upgrade the human experience. Nanotechnology has the potential to help biohackers in a variety of ways, including:

1. **Disease Prevention and Treatment**: Nanotechnology allows for a more precise approach to medicine, from creating nanoscale drugs that target specific cells to designing nanorobots capable of directly manipulating cellular mechanisms. This has the potential to improve medical treatments, reduce side effects, and even prevent diseases before they occur.
2. **Enhanced Senses and Cognitive Abilities**: The development of nanotechnology-based brain implants could allow users to expand their cognitive abilities, such as increasing memory capacity, improving learning rates, or even enabling mind-to-mind communication. Additionally, nanotechnology could be used to augment human senses, such as improving vision and hearing or restoring lost senses like taste or smell.
3. **Physical Performance Enhancement**: Nanotechnology advancements may lead to the development of materials and devices that can improve muscle strength, bone density, or cardiovascular performance. Biohackers could potentially leverage these advancements to push their physical limits and optimize the body's performance.
4. **Repair and Regeneration**: Nanotechnology's ability to manipulate materials on a molecular level has the

potential to enable the development of advanced regenerative therapies. Such therapies could promote rapid healing, replacement of lost or damaged tissue, and even facilitate the growth of new organs.

5. **Age Reversal and Life Extension**: Nanotechnology could play a vital role in research on aging and longevity. Modified nanoscale particles, such as liposomes and nanoparticles, can improve the bioavailability and functionality of age-fighting antioxidants, hormones, or other compounds. Additionally, nanotechnology has the potential to directly repair cellular damage that accumulates with age, thereby slowing or even reversing the aging process.

9.1.3 Key Advancements in Nanotechnology and Biohacking

As nanotechnology continues to progress, a plethora of innovations are emerging with the potential to revolutionize biohacking. Some of these key advancements include:

1. **Nanobots**: Nanorobots, or nanobots, are microscopic machines that are being developed to deliver drugs to specific cells, repair tissue damage, or directly manipulate cellular mechanisms. In the future, advanced nanobots could even have the potential to perform surgeries or monitor vital signs from within the body.

2. **Neural Interfaces**: Scientists are developing nanotechnology-based neural interfaces to create connections between the human brain and external devices, such as computers or prosthetic limbs. These interfaces could enable users to control technology with their thoughts, as well as improve learning rates or increase memory capacity.

3. **Smart Dust**: Smart dust is a concept that involves the development of tiny, wireless sensors capable of recording and transmitting data. In the context of biohacking, these small sensors could be used to track fitness and health data, monitor vital signs, or even provide augmented reality experiences that enhance daily life.
4. **Soft Robotics**: Soft robotics is an interdisciplinary field that combines biology, materials science, and nanotechnology to create robots with flexible, elastic, and responsive components. Soft robots could be used in a biohacking context to assist with muscle strength and flexibility or assist in tissue regeneration and healing.

As we forge ahead in our journey to understand and augment the human body, the future is seemingly limitless with the promise of nanotechnology. The ability to manipulate materials and systems at the molecular scale holds the potential to push the boundaries of biohacking, resulting not only in optimized health and performance but also in the integration of the human body with technology in ways we cannot yet fully imagine.

9.4 Nanotechnology: The Tiny Revolution Changing Your Body from Within

In the world of biohacking, advancements in technology continuously demonstrate potential to enhance the human body's performance in ways beyond our imagination. One of these cutting-edge technologies that have garnered significant attention over the past few years is nanotechnology.

9.4.1 What is Nanotechnology?

Nanotechnology is the manipulation and control of matter at the nanometer scale (i.e., around 1 to 100 nanometers). To give you some perspective, a sheet of paper is about 100,000 nanometers thick. Nanotechnology has promising applications in various fields such as medicine, energy production, and electronics, among others.

9.4.2 Nanotechnology in Biohacking

Biohackers have been increasingly turning to nanotechnology to optimize their health and enhance their body's performance. In this subsection, we'll explore some of the exciting and promising applications of nanotechnology in biohacking:

1. Drug Delivery Systems: One of the greatest challenges in medicine is ensuring that drugs reach their target efficiently while limiting side effects. Nanotechnology has shown promise in the development of smart drug delivery systems able to target specific cells, tissues, or organs more effectively. This results in enhanced therapeutic effects while minimizing the unwanted side effects of the medications. These drug delivery systems could be particularly useful for biohackers, who frequently experiment with different substances to boost their mental and physical performance.

2. Nanobots for Diagnosis and Treatment: Breakthroughs in nanotechnology have paved the way for nanobots - tiny machines capable of navigating our bodies' circulatory and lymphatic systems to perform various tasks. These nanobots could potentially be programmed to diagnose diseases, deliver drugs, or even perform small-scale surgeries on a cellular level. While still experimental, some biohackers are excited about the potential of using nanobots to optimize and enhance their bodies.

3. Tissue Engineering and Regeneration: Nanotechnology has been instrumental in the development of biomaterials that can mimic the functions of native tissues. These materials can be used to engineer new organs or tissues, offering new possibilities for regeneration and healing, in both an aesthetic or functional sense. For example, nanotechnology-based wound dressings can help accelerate the healing process or reduce scarring, while engineered tissues can someday replace damaged muscles or organs.

4. Boosting Athletic Performance: Nanotechnology also has potential applications in enhancing human athletic performance. By using nanomaterials to create lighter, stronger, and more flexible materials, engineers can design clothing, footwear, and equipment that can help athletes (or biohackers seeking to improve their physical performance) train and compete more efficiently.

5. Brain-Computer Interfaces (BCI): New developments in nanotechnology have also advanced the field of BCI. Nanomaterials are being used to create electrodes that can be implanted directly into the brain, enabling the direct integration of electronic devices with our nervous system. In the future, this could allow for more precise control and feedback from devices such as robotic limbs or even systems that could enhance cognitive functions.

9.4.3 Ethical and Safety Concerns

As with any technological advancements, particularly those involving modification or manipulation of the human body, several ethical and safety concerns arise. One concern revolves around the potential long-term health effects of introducing nanoscale materials into our bodies. Current research on this subject remains inconclusive, leading some biohackers to approach nanotechnological applications with caution.

Another significant ethical concern stems from the potential societal implications of widespread nanotechnology use as an enhancement in biohacking. If these technologies become available only to those who can afford them or are willing to take the risk, it could result in an inequitable distribution of benefits and resources, creating a divide between those who are "enhanced" and those who are not.

9.4.4 Conclusion

Despite the challenges and concerns, nanotechnology undeniably offers a world of opportunities and applications for biohackers looking to push the boundaries of human performance. As our understanding of this field grows and we continue making technological strides, we can only begin to imagine the limitless potential that nanotechnology will have in enhancing the human body from the inside out.

10. Beyond the Blueprint: Cultivating Lifelong Health and Continuous Growth

10. Beyond the Blueprint: Cultivating Lifelong Health and Continuous Growth

When you've begun to master the techniques in "Body by Design," you'll start to see dramatic differences in your health, fitness, mental sharpness, and overall well-being. Your next challenge is to push past the limits of the biohacker's blueprint and forge a lifelong path of continuous growth and self-improvement. With the foundation laid out in this book, you're ready to explore beyond the boundaries of your comfort zone and unlock your body's full potential.

10.1 Developing a Growth Mindset

"In a growth mindset, people believe that their most basic abilities can be developed through dedication and hard work—brains and talent are just the starting point." - Carol S. Dweck

The first step in cultivating lifelong health and continuous growth is to adopt a growth mindset. Believing that your abilities and intelligence can be improved through effort, curiosity, and mastery sets the stage for sustained development. By embracing a growth mindset, you recognize that every failure, setback, or obstacle is an opportunity for learning and growth. This determination to evolve and adapt will help you push past plateaus and continue challenging yourself throughout your journey.

Some strategies to cultivate a growth mindset include:

- Setting specific and challenging goals
- Embracing failure as a learning opportunity
- Celebrating progress and small wins
- Actively seeking feedback and applying it constructively
- Constantly seeking new techniques or strategies to enhance your skills

10.2 Continuous Learning and Experimentation

Your journey to optimal health is, first and foremost, a learning experience. As you move beyond the basics outlined in this book, you'll encounter new challenges and opportunities for growth. Pursue ongoing education by reading about new research, attending conferences or workshops, and engaging with like-minded individuals who share your passion for self-improvement.

Stay open-minded and flexible in your approach to your health and wellness journey. Every person's body is unique, and the strategies that work for one individual may not translate perfectly to another. Experiment with different techniques, track your progress, and refine your approach based on the data and insights you gather.

10.3 Building a Support Network

As you embark on your lifelong journey of health and continuous growth, it's essential to surround yourself with supportive, like-minded individuals who share your goals and can offer guidance and encouragement. Build a network of friends, family, colleagues, coaches, and mentors who will challenge you to reach your full potential and motivate you to press forward. Involve yourself in online communities and forums where you can exchange ideas and experiences with other biohackers and fitness enthusiasts.

10.4 Embracing Adaptability

The landscape of health and wellness research is constantly evolving, and the technologies and strategies available to us continue to expand. As you journey further beyond the blueprint, be prepared to adapt to new findings, innovations, and methods. Keep an open mind and maintain your commitment to lifelong learning—your body, mind, and future self will thank you.

10.5 Nurturing Mind-Body-Spirit Connection

As you continue to optimize your health and wellness, recognize the importance of nurturing the connection between your mind, body, and spirit. Developing personal mindfulness practices like meditation, yoga, or deep breathing can help you stay focused and centered amidst the challenges that life throws your way. Cultivate a sense of gratitude and resilience, and foster relationships that enrich your emotional well-being.

10.6 Striving for Balance

In your pursuit of optimal health and growth, it's essential to maintain a sense of balance in your life. Avoid getting caught up in the endless quest for perfection, as this can lead to stress and burnout. Instead, strive for progress over perfection and give yourself permission to take care of your mental health and well-being. Make time for relaxation, hobbies, and social connections and celebrate the progress you make along your journey.

Conclusion: Living a Life of Continuous Growth

As you move beyond the blueprint outlined in "Body by Design," the limits on what you can achieve are bound only by your imagination, dedication, and perseverance. Embrace the challenge to better yourself each day, and cultivate a true passion for learning and self-improvement. With a growth mindset and relentless determination, you hold the key to unlocking your full potential and living a healthy, fulfilling life.

10. Beyond the Blueprint: Cultivating Lifelong Health and Continuous Growth

The journey to optimal health is a never-ending quest for growth and self-improvement. Biohacking, by definition, is the exploration of personal biology to discover the quickest and most effective ways to optimize physical and mental well-being. While the blueprint laid out in this book serves as a solid foundation for a healthy and fulfilling lifestyle, it's essential to remember that true biohackers are always open to learning and adapting their strategies to suit their ever-changing needs and goals.

In this final section, we delve into the various ways you can go beyond the blueprint to cultivate lifelong health and continuous growth. This involves staying informed about emerging research and breakthroughs, developing a growth mindset, embracing habits that promote mental and physical flexibility, and cultivating a strong community of like-minded individuals.

10.1 Staying Informed: Embracing Emerging Research and Breakthroughs

The world of health and wellness is continuously evolving, with new insights, discoveries, and innovations surfacing at lightning speed. As a biohacker, it's crucial to stay abreast of these developments to ensure that your strategies remain effective and up-to-date. Here's how you can keep yourself informed:

1. **Subscribe to reliable sources**: Sign up to receive newsletters, podcasts, or blogs from reputable sources in the fields of health, wellness, and biohacking. Regularly reading or listening to the works of experts can provide insights and inspiration for your pursuits.
2. **Participate in online forums and groups**: Engaging with others who share your passion for biohacking can be an excellent source of information, guidance, and inspiration. Joining online communities such as Reddit, Facebook groups, or dedicated biohacking forums can help you exchange ideas, discuss latest trends, and ask questions.
3. **Attend conferences and workshops**: Participating in live events, such as conferences and workshops, provides an opportunity to learn from leading experts in the fields of health, wellness, and biohacking. Additionally, these events offer valuable networking opportunities, allowing you to connect with fellow biohackers and industry professionals.
4. **Stay skeptical and discerning**: While staying informed is essential, it's equally important to maintain a healthy level of skepticism when encountering new information. Always consider the credibility of the source and ensure the information is backed by solid evidence before incorporating a new tactic into your biohacking toolbox.

10.2 Developing a Growth Mindset: Embracing Personal Change and Adaptability

A key tenet of biohacking is the understanding that there's always room for growth, improvement, and self-discovery.

Developing a growth mindset will not only serve as a driving force in your pursuit of optimal health but also help you navigate life's inevitable challenges and setbacks. Consider the following practices to strengthen your growth mindset:

1. **Embrace change**: Adopting new habits and routines can be challenging, but it's important to remember that change is an essential ingredient for growth. Be open to making adjustments in your strategies as-needed and approach alterations with curiosity, rather than fear or apprehension.
2. **Reframe setbacks as opportunities**: When faced with an obstacle or challenge, instead of seeing it as a failure, consider it an opportunity to learn and grow. Reflect on the situation, identify the lessons to be gained, and utilize that knowledge to make better choices moving forward.
3. **Continuously set new goals**: While it's crucial to celebrate your achievements, never become complacent in your journey towards optimal health. Once you've reached a goal, shift your focus to the next opportunity for growth and personal development.

10.3 Fostering Flexibility: Strengthening Mental and Physical Resilience

Adaptability is a key component of a successful biohacking journey. The more resilient and flexible you are, both mentally and physically, the better equipped you'll be to handle challenges and ultimately reach your desired level of health and wellness. Here are some ways to foster your flexibility:

1. **Prioritize regular movement**: Integrating various types of movement into your daily routine, such as

stretching, yoga, or dynamic exercises, can help to increase your physical flexibility and resilience.
2. **Develop emotional intelligence**: Cultivate self-awareness, practice empathy, and improve your communication skills to become more adaptable in social situations and better equipped to manage stress and anxiety.
3. **Meditate**: Regular meditation practice can significantly enhance mental clarity, focus, and resilience. By cultivating a mindful approach to life, you'll be better equipped to navigate challenges, adapt to new situations, and maintain focus on your goals.

10.4 Cultivating a Supportive Community: Connect with Like-minded Individuals

Embarking on your biohacking journey solo can be daunting and isolating. Establishing a network of like-minded individuals can provide emotional support, motivation, and accountability on your quest for optimal health. Here's how you can build your community:

1. **Participate in local meet-ups and events**: Connect with other biohackers in your area by attending local workshops, seminars, or social events. These gatherings can serve as an invaluable source of inspiration, knowledge, and camaraderie.
2. **Create or join a virtual group**: Establish or join online communities, such as Facebook groups or chat platforms like Slack or Discord, to share your experiences, gain insights, and establish connections with fellow biohackers.
3. **Invite friends and family to join you**: Your loved ones can be an invaluable source of support and motivation. Encourage them to participate in your

biohacking pursuits, extend an invitation to join you on your journey, and share the benefits of embracing a healthy, optimized lifestyle together.

In conclusion, cultivating lifelong health and continuous growth as a biohacker involves staying informed about emerging trends, embracing change, fostering mental and physical flexibility, and building a supportive community. By incorporating these principles into your life, you'll be well-equipped to continually refine and improve your blueprint for optimal health and to thrive, indefinitely.

10.1 Embracing the Journey: Developing a Growth Mindset for Lasting Wellness

Achieving optimal health and maintaining it throughout your life is not a destination, but a journey. It requires ongoing commitment to learning, resilience when facing setbacks, and adaptability to evolving scientific knowledge and personal changes. Biohacking offers you the tools, technologies, and strategies to help you become the architect of your well-being. In this section, we will explore the importance of cultivating a growth mindset, staying informed, and continually challenging yourself to surpass your own limitations, as you build the most robust, resilient, and radiant version of yourself.

10.1.1 Cultivating a Growth Mindset: The Power of Possibility

A growth mindset is a belief in your own capacity to develop, change, and improve. This concept, introduced by psychologist Carol Dweck, suggests that individuals who possess a growth mindset see their abilities, intelligence, and even their bodies as something that can be continually honed and enhanced. As a biohacker, embracing a growth mindset is essential, as it allows you to:

- Recognize that you have the power to change your habits, physiology, and even genetic expression.
- Seek out challenges and enjoy the process of self-experimentation.
- Treat setbacks as opportunities to learn, refine, and iterate on your strategies.
- View new information and scientific advances as exciting discoveries that can help you further optimize your health.

To foster a growth mindset, remind yourself of the immense potential hidden within your biology. From your brain's neuroplasticity to your body's ability to regenerate and repair, never underestimate the transformative power that lies within you.

10.1.2 Staying Informed: The Evolving Landscape of Biohacking and Health Science

The field of biohacking and health science is advancing at a dizzying pace, with new research, tools, and techniques being introduced almost daily. To make the most of these cutting-edge developments and continuously refine your blueprint for optimal health, it is crucial to stay informed and keep learning. Some strategies to stay abreast of the latest ideas and discoveries include:

- **Subscribing to newsletters, podcasts, and YouTube channels** from reputable biohacking and health experts: Keep up to date with the evolving

conversation surrounding health and wellness by following thought leaders in the field.
- **Attending conferences, workshops, and seminars**: Stay connected to the biohacking community, share knowledge and experiences, and learn from experts in a live environment.
- **Participating in online forums and social media groups**: Engage with a global community of biohackers who share your passion for optimal health, discuss your experiences, and learn from one another.

Additionally, make time to review your own health and wellness strategies regularly. As you gather new information and insights, you may discover previously overlooked techniques or new technologies that could enhance your health journey. Be open to experimentation and continuously refining your biohacking blueprint to maximize your wellness potential at every stage of your life.

10.1.3 Challenge Yourself: Breaking Boundaries and Setting New Standards

As you progress on your health journey and successfully implement positive changes to your daily routines, nutrition, and overall well-being, you will likely start experiencing the benefits of your hard work. However, it's crucial to avoid complacency and continuously seek new ways to challenge both your mind and body. Engaging in regular mental and physical challenges allows you to:

- Unlock untapped reservoirs of resilience and ability.
- Break through plateaus and stagnation, ensuring continued progress.
- Build upon your successes and establish an upward spiral of personal growth and wellness.

Some examples of how you might challenge yourself and establish new benchmarks for health and performance include:

- Pushing your body through progressively more difficult physical activity, such as increasing your workout intensity or exploring new training modalities.
- Handling stress proactively by engaging in regular relaxation techniques such as meditation or breathwork, and finding new methods to manage and even thrive amid life's inevitable stressors.
- Adopting a proactive approach to mental health, cognitive agility, and mindset by seeking out opportunities for continued learning, creative expression, and emotional development.

Remember that the journey toward optimal health and wellness is an ongoing and ever-evolving pursuit. By fostering a growth mindset, staying informed, and continually challenging yourself, you can transcend limitations, unlock your full potential, and cultivate lifelong health and vitality.

Embracing the Learning Mindset for Lifelong Health

A vital component of biohacking and building the body by design is cultivating a mindset of continuous learning and growth. With the world of health and wellness continually evolving, it is essential to stay current and adaptable to new findings and techniques. The human body is incredibly complex, and there is no one-size-fits-all solution. Embracing a learning mindset ensures that you remain an active participant in your health journey and can respond to new information as it becomes available.

Importance of a Learning Mindset

The learning mindset is characterized by curiosity, openness to new ideas, and a willingness to experiment and iterate. Cultivating a learning mindset has numerous benefits for your health and wellbeing:

1. **Staying informed**: By continuously seeking information, you can stay up-to-date on the latest insights and advances in wellness technology, allowing you to make the best possible decisions for your health.
2. **Harnessing personal experience:** Building self-awareness and understanding how your body responds to different types of biohacks in real-time is paramount. A learning mindset empowers you to leverage your experiences and refine your strategies for success.
3. **Reduced risk of complacency**: Becoming stagnant in your approach to health can lead to a plateau or even a decline. Continuously learning and adapting keeps you motivated and striving for improvement.
4. **Enhanced resilience**: Having a learning mindset enables you to adapt and overcome setbacks, minimizing the harm to your health and wellbeing when they occur. It helps you turn challenges into opportunities for growth and learning.

Strategies for Fostering a Learning Mindset

Adopting a learning mindset requires intentionality and practice. Here are some strategies to support your journey:

1. **Embrace a growth mindset:** Recognize that your abilities and health can be developed through dedication and effort. By understanding that you can

grow and change, you will become more open to learning and experimentation.

2. **Practice mindfulness:** Being present in the moment and aware of your body's sensations, emotions, and thoughts can help you identify learning opportunities and encourage curiosity.

3. **Stay humble:** Recognize that there will always be more to learn and that you may not always have the perfect solution. Acknowledge your limitations and be open to input from others.

4. **Cultivate curiosity:** Engage in activities that stimulate your mind and spark new interests. Approach unfamiliar subjects or ideas with a genuine sense of inquisitiveness.

5. **Seek feedback:** Regularly seek input from those around you – friends, family, healthcare practitioners, or other biohackers – to gain perspective on your progress and insights into potential improvements.

6. **Invest in education:** Invest time, money, and energy into learning resources such as books, podcasts, courses, or conferences to expand your knowledge and gain exposure to new ideas and techniques.

7. **Set SMART goals**: Establish Specific, Measurable, Achievable, Relevant, and Time-bound objectives for your health endeavors to monitor progress and encourage growth.

8. **Reflect on successes and failures:** Regularly assess your progress to identify what worked, what didn't, and why. Learn from mistakes and setbacks, viewing them as opportunities to gain valuable knowledge and refine your approach.

Trials and Iterations: Experimenting with different Health Hacks

Biohacking is an ongoing process of experimentation and adjustment. Embrace the learning mindset to approach these trials with enthusiasm, resilience, and openness to learning from each experience.

1. **Research**: Do your due diligence to ensure that any potential biohack or technique is safe, scientifically backed and has a solid rationale before experimenting.
2. **Document**: Maintain a detailed log of your trials, noting your starting point, any changes you're implementing, and tracking your progress over time. This documentation will be valuable in refining your approach and facilitating learning from your experiences.
3. **Listen to your body**: Pay attention to how your body reacts during each trial. Are there any side effects, improvements or unexpected results? Continuously reflect on and learn from these experiences.
4. **Adjust and iterate**: As you experiment with different biohacks, adapt your approach based on the results you observe. Consider trying new techniques or combinations and deconstruct successes to understand the factors contributing to your progress.
5. **Resilience and patience**: Remain patient and persistent as you journey through cycles of experimentation and progress. It can take time to see the results of your efforts, and sometimes setbacks are inevitable. Embrace the learning mindset to use these experiences as a springboard for growth.

By embracing a learning mindset, you set yourself up for lifelong health, resilience and growth. Continuous learning is necessary for staying up-to-date with advancements in health technology and maximizing your potential. Embarking on your biohacking journey is just the beginning – make learning an intentional part of your life to ensure that your body remains by design, not default.

10.1 Embracing the Infinite Game: Health, Learning and Growth as a Lifetime Commitment

To truly harness the power of biohacking and build the body by design, it's essential to understand that success isn't the end goal; it's a continuous, ever-evolving journey. Embracing the mindset of an infinite game, where the purpose is to keep playing, learning and growing, will empower you to continuously improve your health, fitness, and overall well-being for your entire life. In this section, we will explore the most effective strategies for cultivating lifelong health and continuous growth.

10.1.1 The Joy of Learning: How Curiosity Keeps You Healthy

Curiosity and the insatiable hunger for learning are essential traits to thrive in the world of biohacking as these are the primary motivators to research, seek new knowledge, and experiment. Maintaining an open mind and a willingness to learn new things not only leads to better long-term physiological health, but it also enriches cognitive abilities and emotional well-being.

As a biohacker, actively seek new information, techniques, and technologies that can revolutionize the way you approach your health, nutrition, and fitness. Keeping your finger on the pulse of the latest research and breakthroughs will not only improve your skills and knowledge but also boost your motivation to maintain a healthy lifestyle.

10.1.2 Building Your Support Network: The Power of Connection

Embarking on a biohacking journey can feel isolating at times, as your dedication to changing your lifestyle, habits and routines may differ from those around you. Developing a support network of like-minded individuals, mentors, and professionals can help keep you motivated, accountable, and open to new ideas.

Leverage the global biohacking community by attending conferences, meetups, and workshops in your area, or seek out online forums, social media networks, and other digital resources where biohackers share their stories, advice, and research findings.

10.1.3 Incremental Change and Kaizen: The One Percent Improvement

The Japanese philosophy of Kaizen embodies the concept of continuous improvement through small, incremental changes — or what is also known as the "one percent rule." This principle, while simple, can have a profound impact on your life and your quest for optimal health.

Rather than impulsively making drastic changes or pursuing lofty goals, shift your focus to making consistent, manageable improvements to your habits, lifestyle, or routines on a daily basis. It's these incremental changes that compound over time, leading to profound growth and exceptional results.

10.1.4 Mastering Your Mindset: The Importance of Mental Health and Resilience

Of all the variables that contribute to optimal health, mental well-being is perhaps the most critical. A strong, resilient mindset is necessary for weathering the challenges, setbacks, and fluctuations that come with building a body by design.

Through self-awareness, self-compassion, and cognitive training practices like mindfulness, meditation, or journaling, you'll cultivate the mental fortitude to ride out the ebb and flow of life. Moreover, nurturing an unwavering belief in your abilities and self-worth reinforces adaptability and resilience in the face of adversity.

10.1.5 The Power of Ritual and Routine: Developing Discipline and Consistency

Discipline and consistency are two critical components of a successful biohacking journey. These virtues not only keep you on track but also enable you to adapt, experiment, and integrate new knowledge, tools, and approaches into your daily life.

To develop robust discipline, invest time and energy into designing and refining habits, routines, and rituals that align with your long-term goals — whether it's morning meditation, a regular exercise schedule, or a carefully curated nutrition plan. Remember, it's about creating a sustainable and enjoyable lifestyle that supports your physical and mental well-being.

10.1.6 Maintaining Balance and Embracing the Detours: Finding Joy in the Journey

As with any long-term quest, it's important not to lose sight of the bigger picture on the path to optimal health. Stumbles, setbacks, and detours are a natural part of life and allow for invaluable learning and growth opportunities.

Cultivate gratitude, forgiveness, and appreciation for your accomplishments, no matter how small. Embrace the philosophy of "balance in all things" by allotting time to rest, recover, and indulge in your pursuits and passions beyond the realm of biohacking. Remember that the purpose of the infinite game is not to achieve some singular objective, but to revel in the journey itself and continually redefine what it means to live a life of health, vitality, and personal growth.

Copyrights and Content Disclaimers:

AI-Assisted Content Disclaimer:
The content of this book has been generated with the assistance of artificial intelligence (AI) language models like CHatGPT and Llama. While efforts have been made to ensure the accuracy and relevance of the information provided, the author and publisher make no warranties or guarantees regarding the completeness, reliability, or suitability of the content for any specific purpose. The AI-generated content may contain errors, inaccuracies, or outdated information, and readers should exercise caution and independently verify any information before relying on it. The author and publisher shall not be held responsible for any consequences arising from the use of or reliance on the AI-generated content in this book.

General Disclaimer:
We use content-generating tools for creating this book and source a large amount of the material from text-generation tools. We make financial material and data available through our Services. In order to do so we rely on a variety of sources to gather this information. We believe these to be reliable, credible, and accurate sources. However, there may be times when the information is incorrect.
WE MAKE NO CLAIMS OR REPRESENTATIONS AS TO THE ACCURACY, COMPLETENESS, OR TRUTH OF ANY MATERIAL CONTAINED ON OUR book. NOR WILL WE BE LIABLE FOR ANY ERRORS INACCURACIES OR OMISSIONS, AND SPECIFICALLY DISCLAIMS ANY IMPLIED WARRANTIES OR MERCHANTABILITY OR FITNESS FOR ANY PARTICULAR PURPOSE AND SHALL IN NO EVENT BE LIABLE FOR ANY LOSS OF PROFIT OR ANY OTHER COMMERCIAL OR PROPERTY DAMAGE, INCLUDING BUT NOT LIMITED TO SPECIAL, INCIDENTAL, CONSEQUENTIAL, OR OTHER DAMAGES; OR FOR

DELAYS IN THE CONTENT OR TRANSMISSION OF THE DATA
ON OUR book, OR THAT THE BOOK WILL ALWAYS BE
AVAILABLE.

In addition to the above, it is important to note that language
models like ChatGPT are based on deep learning techniques
and have been trained on vast amounts of text data to generate
human-like text. This text data includes a variety of sources
such as books, articles, websites, and much more. This training
process allows the model to learn patterns and relationships
within the text and generate outputs that are coherent and
contextually appropriate.

Language models like ChatGPT can be used in a variety of
applications, including but not limited to, customer service,
content creation, and language translation. In customer
service, for example, language models can be used to answer
customer inquiries quickly and accurately, freeing up human
agents to handle more complex tasks. In content creation,
language models can be used to generate articles, summaries,
and captions, saving time and effort for content creators. In
language translation, language models can assist in translating
text from one language to another with high accuracy, helping
to break down language barriers.

It's important to keep in mind, however, that while language
models have made great strides in generating human-like text,
they are not perfect. There are still limitations to the model's
understanding of the context and meaning of the text, and it
may generate outputs that are incorrect or offensive. As such,
it's important to use language models with caution and always
verify the accuracy of the outputs generated by the model.

Financial Disclaimer

This book is dedicated to helping you understand the world of
online investing, removing any fears you may have about

getting started and helping you choose good investments. Our goal is to help you take control of your financial well-being by delivering a solid financial education and responsible investing strategies. However, the information contained on this book and in our services is for general information and educational purposes only. It is not intended as a substitute for legal, commercial and/or financial advice from a licensed professional. The business of online investing is a complicated matter that requires serious financial due diligence for each investment in order to be successful. You are strongly advised to seek the services of qualified, competent professionals prior to engaging in any investment that may impact you finances. This information is provided by this book, including how it was made, collectively referred to as the "Services."

Be Careful With Your Money. Only use strategies that you both understand the potential risks of and are comfortable taking. It is your responsibility to invest wisely and to safeguard your personal and financial information.

We believe we have a great community of investors looking to achieve and help each other achieve financial success through investing. Accordingly we encourage people to comment on our blog and possibly in the future our forum. Many people will contribute in this matter, however, there will be times when people provide misleading, deceptive or incorrect information, unintentionally or otherwise.

You should NEVER rely upon any information or opinions you read on this book, or any book that we may link to. The information you read here and in our services should be used as a launching point for your OWN RESEARCH into various companies and investing strategies so that you can make an informed decision about where and how to invest your money.

WE DO NOT GUARANTEE THE VERACITY, RELIABILITY OR
COMPLETENESS OF ANY INFORMATION PROVIDED IN THE
COMMENTS, FORUM OR OTHER PUBLIC AREAS OF THE book
OR IN ANY HYPERLINK APPEARING ON OUR book.

Our Services are provided to help you to understand how to
make good investment and personal financial decisions for
yourself. You are solely responsible for the investment
decisions you make. We will not be responsible for any errors
or omissions on the book including in articles or postings, for
hyperlinks embedded in messages, or for any results obtained
from the use of such information. Nor, will we be liable for any
loss or damage, including consequential damages, if any,
caused by a reader's reliance on any information obtained
through the use of our Services. Please do not use our book If
you do not accept self-responsibility for your actions.

The U.S. Securities and Exchange Commission, (SEC), has
published additional information on Cyberfraud to help you
recognize and combat it effectively. You can also get additional
help about online investment schemes and how to avoid them
at the following books:http://www.sec.gov and
http://www.finra.org, and http://www.nasaa.org these are each
organizations set-up to help protect online investors.

If you choose ignore our advice and do not do independent
research of the various industries, companies, and stocks, you
intend to invest in and rely solely on information, "tips," or
opinions found on our book – you agree that you have made a
conscious, personal decision of your own free will and will not
try to hold us responsible for the results thereof under any
circumstance. The Services offered herein is not for the
purpose of acting as your personal investment advisor. We do
not know all the relevant facts about you and/or your
individual needs, and we do not represent or claim that any of

our Services are suitable for your needs. You should seek a registered investment advisor if you are looking for personalized advice.

Links to Other Sites. You will also be able to link to other books from time to time, through our Site. We do not have any control over the content or actions of the books we link to and will not be liable for anything that occurs in connection with the use of such books. The inclusion of any links, unless otherwise expressly stated, should not be seen as an endorsement or recommendation of that book or the views expressed therein. You, and only you, are responsible for doing your own due diligence on any book prior to doing any business with them.

Liability Disclaimers and Limitations: Under no circumstances, including but not limited to negligence, will we, nor our partners if any, or any of our affiliates, be held responsible or liable, directly or indirectly, for any loss or damage, whatsoever arising out of, or in connection with, the use of our Services, including without limitation, direct, indirect, consequential, unexpected, special, exemplary or other damages that may result, including but not limited to economic loss, injury, illness or death or any other type of loss or damage, or unexpected or adverse reactions to suggestions contained herein or otherwise caused or alleged to have been caused to you in connection with your use of any advice, goods or services you receive on the Site, regardless of the source, or any other book that you may have visited via links from our book, even if advised of the possibility of such damages.

Applicable law may not allow the limitation or exclusion of liability or incidental or consequential damages (including but not limited to lost data), so the above limitation or exclusion may not apply to you. However, in no event shall the total liability to you by us for all damages, losses, and causes of action (whether in contract, tort, or otherwise) exceed the amount paid by you to us, if any, for the use of our Services, if any. And by using our Site you expressly agree not to try to hold us liable for any consequences that result based on your use of our Services or the information provided therein, at any time, or for any reason, regardless of the circumstances.

Specific Results Disclaimer. We are dedicated to helping you take control of your financial well-being through education and investment. We provide strategies, opinions, resources and other Services that are specifically designed to cut through the noise and hype to help you make better personal finance and investment decisions. However, there is no way to guarantee any strategy or technique to be 100% effective, as results will vary by individual, and the effort and commitment they make toward achieving their goal. And, unfortunately we don't know you. Therefore, in using and/or purchasing our services you expressly agree that the results you receive from the use of those Services are solely up to you. In addition, you also expressly agree that all risks of use and any consequences of such use shall be borne exclusively by you. And that you will not to try to hold us liable at any time, or for any reason, regardless of the circumstances.

As stipulated by law, we can not and do not make any guarantees about your ability to achieve any particular results by using any Service purchased through our book. Nothing on this page, our book, or any of our services is a promise or guarantee of results, including that you will make any particular amount of money or, any money at all, you also understand, that all investments come with some risk and you may actually lose money while investing. Accordingly, any results stated on our book, in the form of testimonials, case studies or otherwise are illustrative of concepts only and should not be considered average results, or promises for actual or future performance.

tolerance, and the ability to consistently apply the strategies and techniques discussed.